The Diabetes Coach Approach Workbook

Janet Sanders, C.H.C.

authorHOUSE®

AuthorHouse™
1663 Liberty Drive
Bloomington, IN 47403
www.authorhouse.com
Phone: 1-800-839-8640

Published by AuthorHouse 11/25/2014

ISBN: 978-1-4389-5712-8 (sc)

The Diabetes Coach Approach Workbook

Newly Revised & Updated

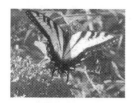

You must be the change you wish to see in the world...

Mahatma Gandhi

Much has happened since I was diagnosed with Type 2 diabetes in 2001 and wrote the original Diabetes Coach Approach Workbook. On a personal level, I have lived with Type 2 diabetes for over 12 years, with many ups and downs and blood sugar highs and lows. Like many of you, I have had times when the stresses of everyday life threatened my ability to maintain normal blood sugars, but because I had a strong program in place, I am happy to say that I made it through.

New medications have been introduced to help manage blood sugars. Some of these drugs are promising, although most still have unwanted side effects. There have been hundreds of new books, seminars, and programs claiming to reverse Type 2 Diabetes. What is interesting is that while there are a number of areas where the medical community and experts agree, there are just as many where there is disagreement, especially when it comes to what to eat.

From moderate approaches that include meat-based protein, whole grains and sugar (in moderation) to totally vegan programs and diets that "forbid" sugar, or grains in any form there is generally no consensus on what to eat.

The truth is that every approach for managing diabetes can point to success stories. Unfortunately, there are also millions of people around the world who have tried and are unable to stick with their "diet" of choice for the long term. And, since I first wrote this book, the diabetes and pre-diabetes statistics are getting worse, not better.

So why an update now?

FIRST: I am more convinced than ever that there is an answer to managing blood sugars, but fad diets and pills or books giving you you more information without telling you how to take action are not the answer.

Side effects aside, when it comes to Type 2 Diabetes, oral medications are Band-Aids that without lifestyle changes usually stop working. Even insulin is not a magic bullet if you are still eating foods that don't support blood sugar management for the long term.

PLEASE NOTE: If you have been prescribed medication, it is ESSENTIAL to follow your doctor's instructions and not to stop taking your medications without discussing this with your physician. Medical care is critical for diabetes and pre-diabetes, but doctors agree that pills alone can't manage high blood sugars. The key is that lifestyle changes have to be part of the overall plan.

With diabetes and pre-diabetes on the rise, experts continue to churn out "diet prescriptions" and the public grabs onto each new diet book hoping that this will be the one that works. Sadly, the majority of dieters get tired of counting, measuring, trying to fit their lifestyle to a rigid menu and feeling deprived. Inevitably, most people quit. For anyone who is an emotional or stress eater, diet plans alone are almost guaranteed to fail.

My goal is to help you ditch the diet mentality and to teach you how to achieve your own blood sugar breakthrough. In short I am going to tell you WHAT you need to do, then I am going to teach you HOW to make the changes needed. I am going to "hold your hand" throughout the process and:

- ❖ demystify the secrets to blood sugar success,

- ❖ unravel the mystery of what to eat, and

- ❖ teach you how to choose foods that let your body function the way it was designed to work so that you can achieve balance and control your blood sugars.

I promise you that figuring out what to eat doesn't have to be so complicated or hard to maintain. That is why I have re-tooled my food plan section to introduce a plan designed to make it even easier for you choose what to eat for good blood sugar control - even on days when life seems to get in the way. The LIVE FREE Food Plan™ provides a foolproof template that combined with the knowledge of how your body works will let you rely less on experts and more on self-knowledge of what works best for you. It is a self-empowering plan that puts you in the driver's seat.

SECOND, after years of researching the many diabetes food plans, my viewpoints have evolved, when it comes to choosing what to eat.

While I still don't believe in "forbidding" any particular food, I am convinced that if you are serious about conquering pre-diabetes and diabetes *for the long term*, eliminating sugar (in all its forms at least 99% of the time) and grain based flour is essential. Likewise, limiting intake of most grains will support blood sugar control and the elimination of cravings. And, this is especially true for stress or emotional eaters.

Many of my clients are very resistant to this idea, I get it. I am sure some of you are already thinking that what I am suggesting is out of the question.

I encourage you to give it a chance. I am going to teach you how to "major" in vegetables, "minor" in healthy proteins of your choice (depending upon whether you are vegan, vegetarian, flexitarian or carnivore) and how to choose a variety of "electives" such as breads that do not contain grain-based flour, healthy fats and oils, sugar alternatives, and low glycemic fruits, that will help you stay satisfied and on track.

You will learn how to make wise choices so that the very occasional detour does not ruin your health or send you back to square one. Most importantly,, you will learn how to make better choices coming from a place of empowerment as opposed to externally imposed rules that eventually get broken.

One of the critical keys to success is finding substitutions and learning how to use 10% of your food choices to keep you feeling liberated from cravings and extreme blood sugar highs and lows. My coaching program will provide you with the information you need to create a food plan that works for you.

The LIVE FREE Diabetes & Blood Sugar Coaching System™ is designed to let you work through the program at a paced that works for you, so some of you may adopt this plan gradually others will embrace it all at once. Regardless of your approach, the end game is the same, and I promise that there will be lots of delicious food to enjoy along the way. If you find that you need extra guidance or support, I have created the "90 Day Blood Sugar

Breakthrough", an on-line/group coaching program designed to be used in conjunction with these materials. You can get more information about how to obtain on-line coaching or join a coaching group at www.diabetescoaching.com.

Some things haven't changed…..

Over 12 years ago an article in the New York Times referred to diabetes as an epidemic "quietly taking its toll." Unfortunately, the one thing that has not changed since I first published The Diabetes Coach Approach Workbook is that there are still millions of people in America and around the world who struggle every day to battle pre-diabetes and diabetes. And unfortunately, the numbers keep rising.

The number of people affected is probably even higher than the statistics indicate because many people don't realize that you don't have to be diabetic to experience blood sugar issues that can have a damaging effect on your body.

❖ Do you ever find yourself at the mercy of unrelenting food cravings? (particularly for sweets, bread, cookies etc.)

❖ Do you experience energy swings that leave you feeling exhausted?

❖ Have you experienced yo-yo weight gain followed by constant dieting?

If you answered yes to any of these questions, it is very likely that roller coaster blood sugar levels and insulin resistance are at the root of the problem.

In fact, today there is a whole new term to describe this phenomenon.

It's called diabesity – which describes the physical symptoms that mark the progression from mild insulin resistance to full-blown diabetes.

And so, this updated version of the Diabetes Coach Approach Workbook is still dedicated to the millions of people all along the "diabetes progression spectrum" in the hope that they will heed the advice of experts who agree that with changes in lifestyle they can avoid becoming another statistic.

If you are diabetic or pre-diabetic, I urge you to take this opportunity to learn about diabetes and to begin a program of self-care. Take a walk. Eat more vegetables. Don't settle for foods that harm you or your family.

If you are a member of the healthcare community, I strongly encourage you to embrace the notion that many patients want to participate in their own healing, and that given the right tools and support they will seek a path towards a better life. Explore different approaches, including inviting health and diabetes coaches to participate in the healing process both as support for your patients and as partners and allies in reaching a common goal: better health for patients and society as a whole.

One thing that still holds true over a decade later, "*One small step at a time, together we can turn the tide*".

Janet Sanders, J.D., Certified Health Counselor, Diabetes Coach
Founder: Great Life, Inc., The Diabetes Coach Approach ™ &
The Blood Sugar & Diabetes Coaching System™
Type 2 Diabetic-September, 2001

Table of Contents

COMING TO TERMS WITH DIABETES

I am a mom, attorney, health counselor, and "type A" personality who likes to get to the heart of a matter and get things done. I don't know how I got this way, but I am not content to take things at face value, and thank God for that. I am also a Type 2 diabetic, and my unwillingness to accept things at face value saved my life.

On the following pages, my story of how I developed diabetes and my journey back to health chronicles how the Diabetes Coaching System™ evolved. If you are a diabetic or pre-diabetic, no doubt you will be able to identify with my experience and become empowered knowing that you are not alone in your thoughts, feelings or daily struggles with diabetes. If you ever feel depressed or burned out by trying to take care of yourself year after year, you are not alone in feeling that way. At those times when you feel particularly challenged by living with diabetes, remember the words of the physician Sir William Osler who almost one hundred years ago remarked: "The way to live a long and happy life is to have a chronic disease and take care of it."

If you are pre-diabetic, even better would be to take the steps now to avoid this chronic disease and continue to take care of yourself well into old age. I have taken the words of Sir William Osler to heart and have found that there is "life" after the diagnosis of diabetes, and it can be a great adventure.

To the friends and relatives of anyone struggling with diabetes, I offer this advice. It is important to grasp that being diagnosed with diabetes is a life changing event, and that your empathy and support are needed in the recovery process. There are many misconceptions about what happens to diabetics after they are diagnosed, both in terms of the course of treatment provided and the type of support needed to successfully keep a chronic illness like diabetes under control. My hope is that my story will shed some light and provide non-diabetics with some new insights on what it is like to be a diabetic.

"It Will Never Happen to Me"

Like many diabetics, I was completely unprepared for the diagnosis. Although diabetes is in my family, I had mentally filed the possibility of getting diabetes under the category of things that would never happen to me.

Actually, it should not have been a surprise. I have struggled with yo-yo weight gain, unmanaged stress and feelings of exhaustion for most of my adult life. The diagnosis came in September 2001, following a familiar pattern of regaining 30 pounds and a particularly stressful period after my father's death. Oddly, although it was a day that changed my life forever, I can't remember the exact date. But, I remember the call from my doctor's office and the circumstances leading up to it as if it were yesterday.

Day One

I had recently started a new job and was feeling extremely tired most of the time. A good friend of mine told me that she had been feeling the same way, and that on her doctor's advice she started taking vitamin B12. "It's really helping" she told me, and as I watched her fly around her office, it certainly seemed to be doing the trick. So, I made an appointment with my doctor, confident that some extra sleep and vitamins would fix me right up. After a short visit and several vials of blood work, my doctor sent me on my way. He told me not to worry and that his office would call me in a few days with the results. When the call came, I was completely thrown off guard by the news.

Just home from work, I was in my kitchen getting ready to have my daily fix of tea and "carbohydrates" before cooking dinner. When the phone rang and the nurse from my doctor's office was on the other end of the line, I wasn't the least bit worried. Although I had experienced some health scares throughout my life, my fears had always been calmed by the words "your tests are normal, everything is fine." I took it for granted that this call would not be any different.

My confidence was buoyed by the sound of the nurse's voice on the other end of the line. I thought, if it was bad news, the doctor would have called me himself. But, it was the nurse who on this day, without any warning, told me that I had diabetes.

I remember feeling disoriented, as if I hadn't heard her correctly. I broke into a cold sweat, and I felt my heart racing. I wanted to tell her that this simply was not possible. A little less than a year before I had applied for a life insurance policy and although my triglycerides were pretty high, my blood sugar levels were normal. If ignorance is bliss, it occurred to me that the previous year must have been pretty darn blissful. Like so many diabetics, I had blindly wandered through the year oblivious to the warning signs that were propelling me towards physical disaster. When my body finally became clinically ill I wondered, "How could this have happened?"

For an attorney that is supposed to have a fairly high level of intelligence and usually in control of my circumstances, all of a sudden I felt extremely stupid and way out of my league. I had no idea what I was supposed to do with this information or what would happen next. Sensing my discomfort, the nurse softened her voice and said "don't worry, a lot of people have diabetes."

I had known this nurse for many years and I think she could feel the tears that were falling on the other end of the line. She tried to reassure me that everything would be fine. Clearly, she did not know that my world was turning upside down, while hers was still perfectly intact. For no logical reason, I wanted to lash out at her and make her feel as bad as I did. But, instead, I asked her what I needed to do next. As she had told so many new diabetics before me, she replied, "you need to come into the office tomorrow for a follow up visit, and the doctor will tell you what to do."

I hung up the phone, turned off the stove and went upstairs to have a good cry. I wasn't sad, I was incredibly angry. Up in my bedroom I just started screaming, "I'M SO MAD, I'M SO PISSED OFF, I DON'T WANT TO HAVE DIABETES!" Finally, exhaustion took over and my screams gave way to sobbing, sobbing to quiet weeping. My poor dog didn't know what was wrong. He ran up the steps, jumped onto the bed and licked my face trying to get me to cheer up. I curled up in a ball with my furry friend and a sense of calm took over.

I don't think the anger ever really goes away, especially once you learn that diabetes is something that could have been avoided. But, my crying jag over, I made a decision not to be a victim and to take control of my situation. Then, I picked myself up, went downstairs to finish making dinner, and for the last time I ate whatever I wanted. And so began my diabetes odyssey and the birth of the Great Life Coaching programs.

A New Beginning

The next day, I left my doctor's office armed with medication, the phone number of a dietician, and very little information about what to do next. With the words "no cure" ringing in my ears, I knew that I needed a plan. More than that, I knew with certainty that I did not want to lose my toes, my kidneys, my eyesight, or my quality of life, and that I was not going to allow these dreaded complications to happen to me. With few real answers for how I was going to bring my blood sugars, weight, high triglycerides and newly forming retinopathy under control, I knew that I had to find a way to do things differently in order to reclaim my health.

Searching for guidance, I started my "quest" in the library and bookstores. I learned that the experts agree that weight loss, exercise, and a healthy diet can help to control the effects of diabetes. For those with high risk factors, early awareness coupled with lifestyle changes can prevent or delay the onset of diabetes.

I also discovered that when it came down to providing dietary guidelines, there were lots of books offering advice on what to eat, but the crazy thing was that much of the advice was conflicting. I carried a pile of books to a table in the bookstore and started going through them.

By closing time my head was spinning. The only thing I knew for sure was that something was wrong with this picture. Nobody seemed to be able to agree on anything, and I was more confused than when I started. The biggest shock to me was that when I browsed through diabetic cookbooks, recipe after recipe had sugar in it. My gut told me that eating sugar didn't make any sense. How could eating a substance that my pancreas cannot handle and that was robbing my body of nutrients in order to metabolize it possibly be a good idea?

Being new to all of this, I decided not to make any snap judgments. The only common thread that I could clearly see was that eating more whole foods and vegetables and exercising would start me on the road to health. But, learning what to eat wasn't going to be enough. I had tried almost every diet out there and lost the same 30 pounds several times in my lifetime. Without a doubt, I knew that the secret to beating diabetes would not just be in the food. So, this time I took a different path and learned that the most important thing I needed to change was my mind, and by doing that, I changed my life and regained my health and well-being.

Stopping the Insanity

How did I turn my health around? The first challenge was finding a model for making effective and lasting lifestyle changes. In the Unites States, health and wellness is a trillion dollar industry. Yet, for all our efforts, the rise in diabetes, obesity and other types of chronic illness suggests that something is amiss. One definition of insanity is ***doing the same thing over and over again and expecting different results***.

As I started putting my plan together, it was clear to me that there was plenty of information available telling diabetics WHAT to do. But there was not a whole lot of guidance on HOW to implement the changes that are necessary to control diabetes or how to deal with the emotional impact of the day to day struggle with the disease.

What I needed to develop was a framework for implementing change and bringing my diabetes under control. I went back to the bookstore, but this time I did not look in the diabetes section. I was in search of information that would help me successfully navigate change. I wanted to develop a program that would empower me and other individuals to:

❶ Think about health in a new way,

❷ Gain the information needed to make informed lifestyle decisions, and

❸ Successfully implement lifestyle changes that will last a lifetime.

After a few hours of searching I found two books that ignited my transformation. The first was a book called "Transitions, Making Sense of Life's Changes" by William Bridges, and the second was a little gem of a book called "The Art of Getting Well" by David Spero. I devoured their contents and applied this new knowledge to the planning techniques that I had mastered as an attorney, consultant and technical change management consultant.

I spent the better part of year working with a doctor specializing in integrative medicine, taking cooking classes, studying nutrition, and developing coaching techniques, while at the same time applying the principles I was learning to my own recovery. I then attended the Institute of Integrative Nutrition and received my certification as a Health Counselor which included joint credits from Columbia University's Teachers College. The end result was a program of coaching and education that would provide the practical tools and information pre-diabetics need in order to prevent full blown diabetes and that would encourage diabetics to take charge of their health and control their blood sugars.

In a nutshell, I started by making a full and honest assessment of my situation and identifying a vision of what I wanted my health and life to be in the future. I worked on letting go of behaviors and habits that were keeping me stuck in the past. Then, one step at a time I implemented a plan of action that would enable me to reach my personal lifestyle goals.

My recovery led me to develop the LIVE FREE Blood Sugar & Diabetes Coaching System™, an innovative program consisting of **coaching**, **education**, and **support** designed to teach individuals how to make healthy lifestyle changes and bring their life back into balance. The story of my healing journey that inspired this program is described on the following pages.

Conquering Diabetes One Step at a Time

> **The World Health Organization (WHO) defines health as a state of complete physical, mental, social and spiritual well-being, and not merely an absence of disease or infirmity.**

With this in mind, I started the process of getting well by creating a vision of what I wanted my health to look like in the future. I knew I wanted more than to get my blood sugars under control. That was critical, but I also wanted to get my energy back and to regain my quality of life I wanted to have **VIBRANT** health, and I made a decision to build a solid foundation based upon six key components of physical, mental and spiritual well-being. These "pillars of vibrant health" are shown in the diagram below.

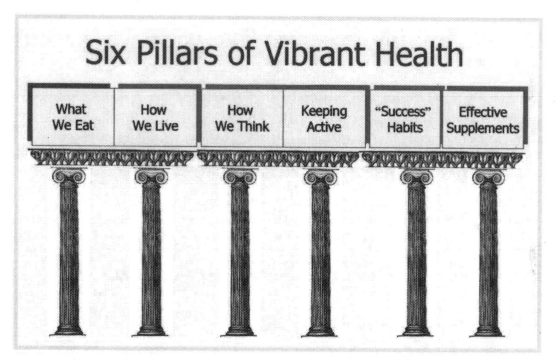

Six Pillars of Vibrant Health

| What We Eat | How We Live | How We Think | Keeping Active | "Success" Habits | Effective Supplements |

My Journey Back to Health

First, I educated myself about diabetes and took responsibility for changing my lifestyle. I took stock of where I was physically and mentally. I asked myself hard questions about how I had been living, what thoughts and behaviors stood in my way, and what new habits I wanted to establish. Then I set goals for what I wanted to accomplish. With my vision and goals in hand, I identified a series of action steps to implement my plan.

Second, I developed a support network of individuals who could help me reach my goals. This included a family doctor with a background in integrative medicine, an endocrinologist, and a nutritional coach who helped me develop diabetes friendly versions of my favorite foods and recipes. With a clear picture of my condition and the support of my team I felt confident that I could turn my health around.

Third, I made a commitment to change my diet and set a goal to lose 30 pounds. I cut out refined, highly processed food products and sugar, added more fiber and vegetables, watched both my fat intake and portion sizes and drank 8 glasses of water a day. As a general guideline, I try to eat a diet with a strong foundation in unprocessed plant foods, primarily those that are low on the glycemic index, with the addition of high quality fats and proteins.

In the beginning, I experimented with different foods by measuring my glucose levels after eating to see the effects of different ingredients. Monitoring my blood sugar on a daily basis is a critical tool to keep my glucose levels under control. Mentally, once I was able to let go of the anger over what I thought I was giving up and started being grateful for the positive me that was emerging, the new way of eating began to get easier and the weight started coming off.

Fourth, I got moving. Exercise provides a number of benefits including clearing the blood of glucose, increasing insulin sensitivity, and improving cardiovascular health. Early on my doctor told me to think of exercise as my insulin, and I took her words to heart. I exercise at least 30 minutes every day, incorporating activities that fit my lifestyle into my exercise routine.

Fifth, I added a program of targeted nutritional supplementation to my lifestyle program. My research convinced me that in conjunction with diet and exercise, adding certain supplements would help with glucose metabolism and insulin sensitivity and could reverse some of the complications I was already experiencing, such as tingling and intense itching in my legs and feet.

After several weeks of my new diet, exercise and the addition of key supplements, my energy returned, the tingling and itching disappeared, my glucose levels normalized, my triglyceride levels went down and I began losing weight. Vitamins and nutrients that I have found most helpful include: Alpha Lipoic Acid, GTF Chromium, Magnesium, Vitamin D, Banaba Leaf, Garcinia Cambogia (HCA), Vanadium, a formulation of antioxidants, and essential fatty acids.

Sixth, I made my recovery a priority and started actively managing the stress in my life. I learned that stressful situations will not go away just because I have diabetes, but discovered that walking, breathing exercises, hobbies, meditation, and getting enough sleep are all excellent aids in keeping stress under control.

Determined to manage my diabetes with lifestyle adjustments and minimal medication, one step at a time I consistently did whatever was needed to get my blood sugar levels under control. The end result has been an opportunity to improve my overall health. In six months I lost over thirty pounds, reduced my medication and normalized my blood sugars. Years later my weight and my blood sugars have remain stabilized.

In the next section, you will learn how my personal journey led to the development of the LIVE FREE Blood Sugar & Diabetes Coaching System™ and why health coaching is a missing link in the fight against diabetes.

THE BIRTH OF THE LIVE FREE BLOOD SUGAR & DIABETES COACHING SYSTEM™

The Diabetes Epidemic

I'm certainly not the only person who has managed to get their diabetes under control. There are many diabetics throughout America and around the world who successfully manage their diabetes, both with and without medication. On the other side of the coin, there are thousands (perhaps millions) more who are unable to prevent the onslaught of this disease and who suffer from a myriad of complications. Consider the following statistics:

❖ **An estimated 26 million Americans have diabetes.** In addition, an estimated 79 million have pre-diabetes. The majority, 90-95%, have Type 2 diabetes. (An estimated 7 million of these Americans are not aware of their diabetes.)

❖ **Today, diabetes causes more deaths a year than breast cancer and aids combined.** In 2013 the U.S. Department of Health and Human Services reported that Diabetes was the 7th leading cause of death, as reported on death certificates in the Unites States. This number accounts for deaths directly attributed to diabetes. It does not account for deaths indirectly caused by diabetes, and if current trends continue, yearly deaths due to diabetes could triple by 2025. (It is also the leading cause of new cases of blindness, kidney failure, and lower-extremity amputations.) 2 out of 3 people with diabetes die from heart disease and stroke.

❖ **According to the American Obesity Association, an estimated 120 million adults are either overweight or obese**. 85% of people with Type 2 diabetes are overweight or obese. As Jeffrey Koplan, former Director for the CDC notes: "…With obesity on the rise, we can expect the sharp increase in diabetes rates to continue. Unless these dangerous trends are halted, the impact on our nation's health and medical care costs will be overwhelming."

❖ **Centers for Disease Control estimate that by the year 2050, the prevalence of diabetes will increase by 165%**. As many as 1 in 3 Americans will have diabetes in 2050 if present trends continue. Dr. Martin Silink, the President of the International Diabetes Federation warns, "Diabetes is one of the biggest health catastrophes the world has ever seen. The diabetes epidemic will overwhelm health care resources everywhere if governments do not wake up now and take action."

Perhaps the most frightening trend is the rise in Type 2 diabetes in children. Before the mid 1990's it was rare for pediatric centers to diagnose children with Type 2 diabetes. Today over 3,000 youth are newly diagnosed with type 2 diabetes annually. It is now estimated that **without a change in childhood obesity rates, 1 out of every three children born today and in the future will be diagnosed with Type 2 diabetes at some point in their lifetime**.

Faced with fast food, super-size snacks and sodas, an overabundance of highly processed foods, less physical activity and an increasingly fast paced and stressful environment, it is small wonder that the most vulnerable in our society are falling prey to Type 2 diabetes. Something is gravely wrong.

If it is true that it takes a village to raise a child, what are we as the villagers doing to turn the tide and provide an infrastructure that doesn't cause permanent harm to our children?

Unfortunately we are not doing enough. Ironically, we are a nation obsessed with wellness. The bookstores are full of books about conquering diabetes, cooking for diabetes, and warning about the current diabetes crisis. If information were the key to optimal health, by all rights we should be the healthiest nation on the planet. Yet as the statistics show, the number of Americans with diabetes, obesity and other chronic diseases continues to spiral upwards with no end in sight.

Why Do Some Succeed Where Others Fail?

There are many diabetics who refuse to let diabetes destroy their health and well-being. There are also many pre-diabetics or people with risk factors such as obesity who turn their health around. They are the success stories.

Many others slowly spiral into an unhealthy state and suffer massive complications and ultimately death. So, why do some people succeed at managing their diabetes while others find it almost impossible? What is the common denominator among people who are able to get their diabetes under control?

The answer does not lie in science, pills or the latest diet plan. People who succeed in changing their lifestyle have the following in common.

❖ **Attitude**: They are willing to do what it takes to make necessary changes.

❖ **Vision**: They have a plan of action, and they follow up that plan with consistent actions that lead them towards health.

❖ **Support**: They have support from various sources, including health care providers, organizations or someone who can guide them as to how to make changes that they can incorporate into their daily lives.

❖ **Resources**: They have access to tools and resources such as medical care, glucose monitors, medication, healthy food, and other resources needed to promote blood sugar control.

❖ **Courage**: Most importantly, they have the will and the courage to take their lives back from the cultural influences that are geared and designed to make and keep them sick.

It is only common sense that any plan or program aimed at breaking the diabetes cycle needs to take into account the factors that will foster success.

Unfortunately, providing information, insulin and pills is easy. Changing human behavior is not.

If the good news is that diabetes can be managed by making needed lifestyle changes, the bad news is that the current medical system is not set up to help individuals to successfully prevent and manage this disease. As we will learn in the next section, the inability of our society to get a handle on the diabetes epidemic affects us all.

The Hidden Costs of Diabetes

The costs of diabetes are staggering both in terms of human suffering and economics.

In 2013 it was estimated that the total annual economic cost of diabetes in the United States was $245 billion, up from $174 billion in 2007. This includes $176 billion in direct costs and $69 billion in indirect costs (lost workdays, restricted activity days, mortality, and permanent disability).

If you are not diabetic and think that diabetes has nothing to do with you, think again. Because of its chronic nature, the severity of its complications and the means required to control them, diabetes is a costly disease, not only for the affected individual and his/her family, but also for health authorities in the United States and around the world. As the number of people with diabetes grows, the disease takes an ever-increasing proportion of national health care budgets. The costs both in human and economic terms to our society are enormous and will affect us all both today and well into the future.

For most countries, the largest single item of diabetes expenditure is hospital admissions for the treatment of long-term complications, such as heart disease and stroke, kidney failure and foot problems. Many of those are potentially preventable given prompt diagnosis of diabetes, effective patient and professional education and comprehensive long term care.

Yet, as unbelievable as it seems, health and government officials often find it is both easier and more profitable to treat the gross complications of diabetes than to fund education programs. Sadly, many programs that could turn lives around never get off the ground or are discontinued for lack of funding. Even well-funded traditional education programs are not designed for the long term. After the program ends, then what?

Many of my clients attended initial sessions with a doctor prescribed dietician or participated in a traditional diabetes education program. They found that these programs were helpful initially, but with the passing of time, many reverted back to their old habits.

Over time many factors associated with uncontrolled diabetes, including pain, anxiety, inconvenience and generally lower quality of life have a great impact on the lives of individuals and their families. Coupled with a loss of hope, many diabetics fall into a state of depression. They know their life is spinning out of control with frightening consequences at the end of the road, and they don't know how to stop it from happening.

Making matters more complex, many Americans hardest hit by the disease are uninsured or in a financial situation where they can't afford the testing materials, medications, and other treatment needed to stay healthy. Minorities and the poorest segments of our population are at the greatest risk for both the disease and its horrendous complications.

As I will explain in the following sections, all of these factors led to my desire to create an affordable coaching program and virtual on-line coaching center that would be available to anyone seeking to control their blood sugars for the long term.

Underlying Forces: The Food & Health Care Industries

Beyond the issues associated with the individual and political responses to controlling diabetes, there are other underlying forces at work. You might be surprised to learn that diabetes and other chronic illnesses form a financial backbone to both the food and orthodox medical establishment. Should an effective method of reversing the diabetes trend be popularized, the resulting financial impact to the health care industry, several of our tax free foundations and a large part of our food processing industry would be severe.

Pharmaceutical companies provide lifesaving drugs and insulin. (They also provide jobs that support our communities) But, the overall effect of the world wide diabetes epidemic is that they also earn billions of dollars from drugs used to treat diabetes, not to mention the peripheral drugs and procedures needed to treat high cholesterol, heart conditions, and other diabetes complications. This situation creates a profound dilemma.

Many drug companies, medical care providers and a large part of the food industry (that spends billions of dollars promoting and selling foods directly opposed to maintaining good health) would have to greatly change their way of doing business in order to survive a reversal of the diabetes epidemic. Even if only a portion of the 26 million diabetics and 79 million pre-diabetics were able to avoid diabetes or turn their diabetes around, the effect on the health care, pharmaceutical and food industries would be significant. On the other hand, with programs of prevention and control, the savings to individuals and society would be phenomenal both in human and economic terms.

Diabetes Coaching: A New Approach

So now you are starting to understand why treating pre-diabetes and diabetes is such a complex issue.

In order to stem the tide, organizations and individuals must be willing to break out of the matrix of current societal influences and adopt new ways of addressing and managing chronic illness.

> The definition of a "revolution" is a fundamental change in the way of thinking about or visualizing something. This is often referred to as a change in paradigm

When the medical establishment, government and social agencies join together to embrace solutions that address the social issues and empower individuals to make positive changes in their life, the insanity of escalating diabetes and needless suffering will abate on a larger scale.

The plan that I developed to get well was a natural outgrowth of my experiences as a change management consultant. When I was diagnosed with diabetes, my gut reaction was that I could turn my condition around by applying the same principles I had used in the business world to help organizations implement changes in their business processes. It made perfect sense that developing a vision of what I wanted my health to look like in the future followed up by a plan of action for attaining that vision of good health was the place to start. Most importantly, the plan worked.

The problem is getting this message out to the millions of diabetics and pre-diabetics who do not have access to more holistic approaches to diabetes management or who don't have the resources to put a plan into action. Most diabetics/pre-diabetics do not know where to find the long term support and structure that is missing in their treatment or how to change behaviors that are sabotaging their efforts..

With this in mind, I developed a diabetes coaching program to provide anyone struggling with blood sugar issues the blueprint for change that I wish I had been given the minute I walked out of my doctor's office. My mission is to provide individuals struggling with weight, diabetes, pre-diabetes, or related health issues with a practical framework for controlling their blood sugars and regaining their health

Today, I am expanding this program to offer diabetes coaching throughout the United States and the world with the launch of an on-line virtual diabetes coaching center and the "90 Day Blood Sugar Breakthrough" Coaching program. Both are based upon the concepts presented in the LIVE FREE Blood Sugar & Diabetes Coaching System™.

The Synergy of Medical Care and Health Coaching For Lasting Lifestyle Changes

> The blood sugar and diabetes health coaching process is designed to complement and enhance an individual's medical support team by providing information, motivation, and support throughout the lifestyle change process.
>
> It is not a replacement for medical care, and coaching programs can work quite nicely in conjunction with other aspects of diabetes care, such as necessary medications, medically supervised dietary counseling or other educational programs.

The key to coaching's success is that it adds a new dimension to the traditional medical approach which typically focuses on providing medication, some dietary advice and educational programs. The problem with this approach is that patients are left on their own to implement their recovery.

Most medical professionals genuinely want to make a difference in the lives of their patients. Unfortunately, the statistics speak for themselves. The current take some pills, get some information and then "pull yourself up by your bootstraps" plan just isn't working for the majority of people.

The purpose of coaching, in the context of managing diabetes or pre-diabetes, is to help individuals to bring their behaviors and goals in alignment with their vision of health. A good health coaching program will go beyond providing information and will provide concrete tools in order to teach participants how to achieve the results that they desire.

This process addresses the practical aspects of conquering diabetes, including what to eat, how to shop, how to manage daily stress, and how to develop a daily exercise routine. But, more importantly, coaching provides an opportunity for individuals to uncover how their thoughts and behaviors have led them to where they are while also providing the ongoing support and guidance needed to help them to make helpful lifestyle changes.

Most importantly, Health Coaching is About Addressing the Root Cause of Diabetes, Pre-Diabetes and Insulin Resistance and Creating a Life in In Balance

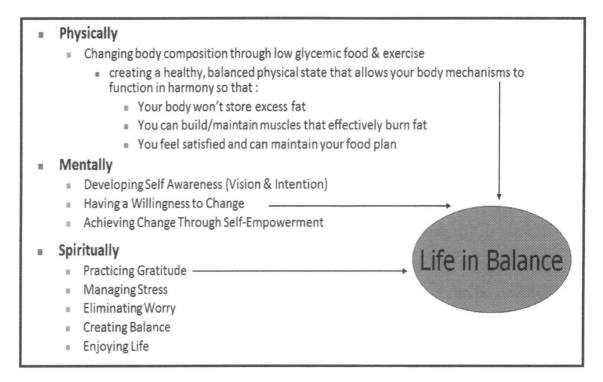

- **Physically**
  - Changing body composition through low glycemic food & exercise
    - creating a healthy, balanced physical state that allows your body mechanisms to function in harmony so that :
      - Your body won't store excess fat
      - You can build/maintain muscles that effectively burn fat
      - You feel satisfied and can maintain your food plan
- **Mentally**
  - Developing Self Awareness (Vision & Intention)
  - Having a Willingness to Change
  - Achieving Change Through Self-Empowerment
- **Spiritually**
  - Practicing Gratitude
  - Managing Stress
  - Eliminating Worry
  - Creating Balance
  - Enjoying Life

Life in Balance

With so much at stake, it only makes sense for diabetics and the medical establishment to take a serious look at how to incorporate motivation and on-going coaching support into the wellness equation.

The good news is that many health organizations throughout the world are embracing new approaches to diabetes care, and the revolution is underway.

One example is a study conducted several years ago by the Design Council in the UK. This study concluded that medical, educational, emotional and motivational support all play a vital part in helping diabetes sufferers to manage their condition effectively.

Case Study: Addressing Diabetes Care in Bolton

Bolton is a large town in Greater Manchester, in North West England with a growing number of diabetics. Health officials were finding that despite the excellent care and support services offered by dedicated facilities such as the Bolton Diabetes Centre, many patients within the community were experiencing difficulty making the lifestyle changes necessary to manage diabetes and avoid the onset of severe complications.

To address these issues, the Open Health project, driven by a team of designers, policy thinkers and social scientists from an organization, The Design Council, came together in order to help transform diabetes care.

The Design Council is a national organization funded by the UK government to promote the use of design led innovation throughout the UK's businesses and public services. One area of focus is the initiation of new thinking about ways to design public services around the needs of people who use them

Working closely with patients and healthcare professionals, the Design Council team concluded that effective self-management of diabetes requires a radical change in behavior. They also found that despite excellent medical and educational support, many diabetics were unable to manage their condition effectively because of a lack of ongoing emotional and motivational support.

Unfortunately, this sort of change is not easily supported by health care institutions where resources are tight and priority must be given to the delivery of medical treatments. The design team came to a realization that the improvement of diabetes care has to be empowered and supported at an individual level.

With this mind, they began to develop a program that would focus on identifying an individual's barriers to change, finding ways to overcome those obstacles and supporting that change into the future.

Ultimately, the team developed the concept of providing a health coach for people with diabetes. The idea behind this solution is that coaches would be able to complement existing educational and medical resources by tackling the issue of chronic disease management from the perspective of the individual.

They developed a concept called "Me2" a system that supports and enables people to live well with diabetes in their everyday lives. It provides a platform for people to co-create care services with professionals that are right for them as individuals. The program also provides access to Me2 coaches that support people in making changes to their lifestyles

Me2 represents a major shift in thinking on the way we approach the management of chronic conditions, and demonstrates how a new organizational model for doing so can be designed to work in practice.

This innovative approach improves a diabetic's chances at success by providing additional tools to support greater control of their disease. For more information about this study go to: http://www.designcouncil.info/RED/health/#B4

Today in the United States, hospitals, clinical groups, government agencies and other organizations are conducting similar types of studies to identify creative approaches to enhancing the medical care of patients with diabetes. Examples include looking at using peer health coaches to help patients with diabetes, and using a care management team to complement the medical care provided by a patient's primary care physician.

As the Bolton team discovered, diabetes presents an opportunity to make positive changes. But, for many diabetics and pre-diabetics, the change process is too overwhelming to tackle without support.

In the following sections we will explore how the LIVE FREE Blood Sugar & Diabetes Coaching System™ empowers diabetics and pre-diabetics (or anyone experiencing blood sugar issues) to make lasting lifestyle changes in order to keep their blood sugars under control.

DIABETES: THE CRISIS AND THE OPPORTUNITY

Seizing the Opportunity for Health

Whether you are someone who has recently been diagnosed with diabetes, pre-diabetes or you have high risk factors for this disease, you have taken a first step in dealing with an unfolding "crisis" in your life.

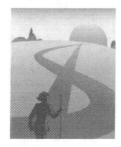 It has been said that a crisis situation has two elements: Danger and Opportunity. The danger feels very real and very scary, and it may not initially occur to you that you can choose to look at this crisis in several ways. One thing is certain, with crisis comes change, and with change comes opportunity. You are about to begin a journey of education and self-exploration that will provide you with the opportunity to change your life.

WHAT YOU DO WITH THIS OPPORTUNITY WILL BE UP TO YOU. When diagnosed with diabetes or pre-diabetes, it is natural to want a "magic pill" to make it go away. Our *fix it fast* culture doesn't promote spending time or energy addressing how we got ill or how to maintain our health into the future. Having diabetes seems hard enough. Taking responsibility for improving your lifestyle may feel overwhelming, and maintaining the level of self-care required to manage diabetes can at times be challenging. But, with support and guidance, facing diabetes does not have to defeat you. In fact, although you might not believe it now, down the road you may find yourself in better shape than you have been in a long time.

Whether you are trying to prevent diabetes or control a diabetic condition, you will learn that neither is about going on a "diet". To the contrary, you will come to understand that controlling blood sugars and maintaining a healthy lifestyle is about making changes that allow your body mechanisms to function in harmony.

When you are in a more balanced, healthy state of well-being, you will feel satisfied and able to maintain your new lifestyle changes. You will learn that in addition to what you eat on a daily basis, there are many components that affect blood sugar levels. Supportive relationships, physical exercise, fulfilling careers, and meaningful spiritual connections all come together to nourish our mind and bodies in ways that significantly affect the healing process.

A WORD OF WARNING: This coaching program is not for everyone.

We often think the job of experts is to give us the answers to our problems. The truth is, when it comes to issues concerning lifestyle, there are no right or wrong answers that fit every person. But there are choices that will lead you towards good health and others that will lead you away from it.

If you are looking for a trendy diet for dealing with diabetes or weight loss you will not find it here. This is not a "diet" program. It is a learning program that will teach you how to make informed choices that support your health and the ability to control your condition. When it comes to eating, you won't have to count, measure or feel deprived because you are going to learn how to eat and live in harmony with the way your body was designed to work.

This program will not propose specific courses of treatment for anyone's particular condition. But, it will provide information that will enable you to create a vision of health along with practical techniques and tools you can utilize to change your lifestyle, achieve your goals, and work effectively with your health care providers.

You will not learn everything there is to know about diabetes in this book. But, you will develop a better understanding about how diabetes and chronic high blood sugar affects your body, and you will learn about resources that can provide you with additional information so that you can continue to learn and grow in your understanding of how to manage your condition.

Coaching Program Overview

The foundation of the LIVE FREE Blood Sugar & Diabetes Coaching System™ is a unique eight point coaching program that provides guidance and support designed to lead you towards your vision of health at all levels: physically, mentally and spiritually.

The self-paced coaching approach will enable you to master the concepts and techniques associated with blood sugar and diabetes control. As you move through the process you will gain:

❖ The confidence to be assertive in your own care,

❖ An understanding of how to use resources to help you explore your options, and

❖ The ability to combine self- knowledge with external information in order to make lifestyle decisions that are right for you.

The coaching program is divided into two main sections. In the first section, "Dynamics of Change" you will become familiar with key concepts that will be used throughout the rest of the coaching program, including:

❖ How grasping the fundamentals of personal change can help you move forward, and

❖ Why understanding basic information about diabetes will help you make lifestyle decisions that will support your vision of health.

The remainder of the book will focus on the **LIVE FREE Blood Sugar & Diabetes Coaching System™**. You will learn how to develop a strategy for managing your condition and how to put your game plan into action.

To clarify and enhance the information in each section, **Key Concepts**, **Reflections** and coaching **Action Steps** are provided throughout the Workbook as described below:

☞ Key concepts (indicated by a Key symbol) are summarized throughout the workbook so that you can find and refer back to them easily.

📖 Reflections are coaching observations that illuminate some of the key concepts presented in the Diabetes Coaching System™.

✎ Action steps are provided to help you put key concepts to work in your coaching program.

Below are some suggestions to maximize the benefits of this program:

❖ **Keep an Open Mind**: Remember, your mind is like a parachute…it only works when it is open. Many of the concepts will be new to you. If you find yourself particularly resistant to making certain changes, use the tools in the course to discover the source of your resistance.

❖ **Take What You Like And Leave The Rest**: The goal of the program is to make sure you have the information, tools and support you need to make and maintain informed lifestyle decisions. Some of the suggestions will be a good fit for you, others may not be. In the end you will need to develop a plan that fits your needs and lifestyle.

❖ **Don't Get Discouraged**: Gaining control of a diabetic or pre-diabetic condition is not easy. There is no race or deadline for you to meet. By working consistently, at your own pace, you will reap the benefits of this program.

❖ **Start a Journal**: Writing and recording your thoughts will help you develop your vision, set goals, and master lifestyle success habits. If you don't already have one, purchase a notebook or journal that you can use to enter your thoughts, respond to exercises, and make notes about items you would like to explore further. Not only does journaling help you gain clarity and reduce stress, but it can also help you stay organized by putting all your thoughts, questions and observations in one place.

❖ **Monitor Your Progress**: Find a tool that you are comfortable with to help you track your daily progress. Recording your blood sugar levels (if you are diabetic), food intake and exercise activities on a daily basis will help you to become more aware of your behaviors while keeping you on track as you work towards your goals.

❖ **Get Structure & Support**: If you find that following the program on your own is difficult for you, one approach is to find a buddy or someone that can provide accountability and support as you move through the process. *My on-line program "The 90 Day Blood Sugar Breakthrough" is designed to complement the written guidelines in this book and to lead participants through the steps in a way that ensures a high level of success. You can learn more about this program at www.diabetescoaching.com.* It is my sincere hope that this program will ignite your journey towards wellness and that for you the Diabetes Coach Approach will be an inspiring force for lasting change.

Are You Ready? LET'S GET STARTED

THE DYNAMICS OF CHANGE

Whatever you can do or dream you can, begin it. Boldness has genius, power and magic in it. Begin it now.

Johann Wolfgang von Goethe

Sometimes change is a welcome challenge. Often it is thrust upon us. Regardless of how the change occurs, everyone responds differently.

There is no "right" way to adapt to and manage a chronic condition. There is no "one size fits all", medication, diet, or exercise plan to solve each individual's diabetic or pre-diabetic condition. *What then is the common denominator among people who are able to get their condition under control?*

An absolute requirement for conquering diabetes or pre-diabetes is a willingness to make lasting lifestyle changes.

❖ The one thing that experts agree on is that early awareness and lifestyle changes can prevent or delay the onset of diabetes. Once diagnosed, making dietary changes, exercising, taking any necessary medications and getting nutritional support can help to control the effects of diabetes and enable individuals with diabetes to live a full life.

❖ The good news is that diabetes is a disease of lifestyle. That means that you can gain control of your self-care and have an impact on the quality of your life. The bad news is that diabetes is a disease of lifestyle. That means that the responsibility for the quality of your life is in your hands.

❖ The most significant factor that will enable you to control your diabetes or pre-diabetic condition long term is your attitude. Diabetes is a prime example of a chronic disease where your behavior is the key to the outcome.

❖ Gaining the knowledge of what changes are needed is not enough. You must be self-motivated to make lifestyle changes coupled with a plan of action.

In his book The Healing Heart, Norman Cousins wrote, "the notion that the focus of healing is lodged with the physician is incorrect. It is lodged with the individual… If [a patient] looks completely outside himself for help, he places an unreasonably large part of the burden on the physician and may retard his own recovery." It is critical to remember, however, that replacing medical care with self-care is not recommended. Complimenting that care with lifestyle improvements can make a big difference.

With support, change provides an opportunity for growth and to attain your dreams. The Diabetes Coaching System™" is designed to incorporate all of the fundamental principles of change so that you will be able to put these principles to work in the context of an action plan. On the following pages, we will take a look at each of these concepts and how they support your ability to conquer diabetes.

Change Your Mind, Change Your Life

The foundation of long term change begins with a shift in thinking coupled with a strategy for implementing new ways of approaching life on a daily basis. The diagram below sets forth the coaching concepts that support this process. These concepts are the foundation of the Diabetes Coaching System™ and are an integral part of what makes the health coaching process successful. Each element is set forth in the one of the points of the six sided star below and described on the following pages, including how each element relates to the steps in coaching program.

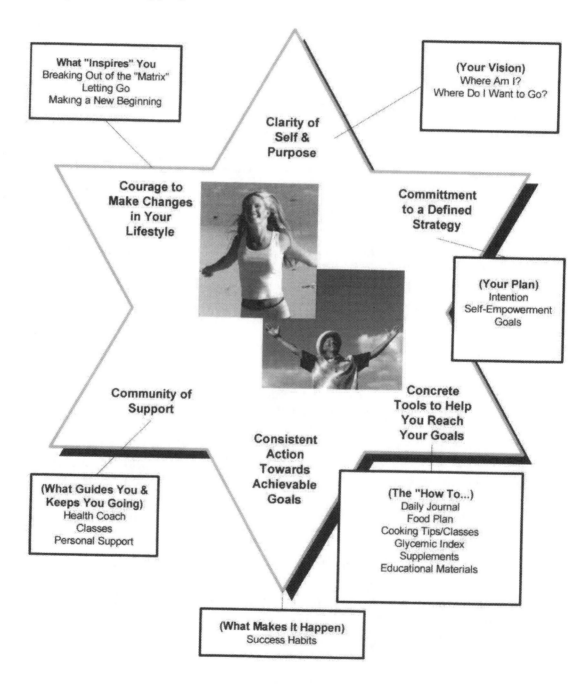

What "Inspires" You
Breaking Out of the "Matrix"
Letting Go
Making a New Beginning

(Your Vision)
Where Am I?
Where Do I Want to Go?

Clarity of Self & Purpose

Courage to Make Changes in Your Lifestyle

Committment to a Defined Strategy

(Your Plan)
Intention
Self-Empowerment
Goals

Community of Support

Concrete Tools to Help You Reach Your Goals

Consistent Action Towards Achievable Goals

(What Guides You & Keeps You Going)
Health Coach
Classes
Personal Support

(The "How To...")
Daily Journal
Food Plan
Cooking Tips/Classes
Glycemic Index
Supplements
Educational Materials

(What Makes It Happen)
Success Habits

CLARITY OF SELF AND PURPOSE: Just because you are ready to move forward does not mean that life will always cooperate. Your job may still be stressful, loved ones need you even when you are bone tired, the food at your cousin's wedding is irresistible, you need to exercise and your back goes out. The motivation that will enable you to reach your goals when obstacles are in your way must come from within, and decisions you make must be made based on your vision of health, unique life goals and bio-individuality.

It is critical that you have the depth of self-knowledge that will enable you to identify behaviors holding you back and to make lifestyle decisions that are right for you. Developing your vision of health, clarifying your physical condition, and monitoring your progress are covered in Steps #1, 3 & 5 of the LIVE FREE Blood Sugar & Diabetes Coaching System™ ("Coaching System"), *Learn About Diabetes, Validate Your Intent with a an Action Plan.& Find Out Where You are and Monitor Your Progress.*

COMMITMENT TO A DEFINED STRATEGY: Most people do not plan to fail. But unfortunately, many times we fail to plan. Having a commitment to a defined set of goals will provide a framework that will assist you in identifying your priorities while keeping you focused and moving forward on a steady path. Goal setting concepts are covered in Steps #3 of the Coaching System, *Validate Your Intent with an Action Plan.*

CONCRETE TOOLS TO HELP YOU REACH YOUR GOALS: The most effective tools for conquering diabetes are a solid food plan, exercise, stress management, nutritional support, and monitoring (in conjunction with any necessary medications/insulin your physician may prescribe). Guidelines and techniques for implementing these tools are discussed in Steps #2 and #5 of the Coaching System, *Implement a Food Plan and Energize Daily with Success Habits.*

CONSISTENT ACTION TOWARDS ACHIEVABLE GOALS: The best plan will not be effective without action to back it up. It is not necessary to make dramatic changes. To the contrary, it's the little things done consistently on a daily basis that will lead you towards your goals. The secrets to changing habits that negatively affect your health and how to implement new Success Habits are discussed in the section "The Secret of Success Habits" in Step #4 of the Coaching System, *Energize Daily with Success Habits.*

COMMUNITY OF SUPPORT: Many people diagnosed with diabetes are lulled into a false sense that their condition is not serious. Don't be fooled. Without treatment, diabetes can be deadly, which is why it is so important to have a circle of support that can provide understanding, encouragement, medical information and a support when times get tough. How to develop a support team that fits your needs is discussed in Step #7 of the Coaching System, *Establish an Ongoing Support System.*

COURAGE TO MAKE CHANGES IN YOUR LIFESTYLE: In her book "Feel the Fear and Do it Anyway", Susan Jeffers notes: "Whenever we face challenges or enter unfamiliar territory or put ourselves into the world in a new way, we experience fear." Moving through that fear requires courage. No matter how small an initial change seems to you, pat yourself on the back for the courage it took to take that step, and keep moving forward with new found confidence that you can conquer whatever blood sugar issues you are facing.. How to work through daily challenges is explored in Step # 6 of the Coaching System, *Reverse Behaviors Sabotaging Your Health.*

Letting Go: The First Step Towards Change

Inherent in every change is an ending. When faced with a changing situation, our reactions run the gamut from *denying*, *ignoring* or *embracing* the fact that an ending has occurred. Often overlooked, an empowering aspect of change is letting of the past. If you can embrace the ending, you can then create the space to embrace a new beginning, and that is one of the great secrets of change.

****

In a sense, endings represent a symbolic death, a parting with the way things were in order to move onto the way they will be in the future. A diagnosis of diabetes or pre-diabetes is a life altering event that requires letting go of the past in order to maintain your health. Although it may seem like taking a step backwards, understanding and appreciating how you feel about what is ending for you will give you both the space and peace of mind to move forward.

Many people get frustrated with this concept. A common reaction is, "I don't want to think about the past, I just want to move on."

There is a world of difference between wallowing in the past and taking some time to acknowledge what is ending for you. This reflection will enable you to clearly identify "where you are" and then move to the next phase, **adapting** and developing a vision of "where you want to go." If you are having trouble implementing lifestyle changes such as foregoing sugar, exercising regularly, managing stress, or cutting back on refined carbohydrates, try working through the exercise on the following page designed to help you move forward.

📖 *Reflections*

Although I now know I didn't develop diabetes overnight, once I was aware that I had this condition I realized that the old me, (the one that ate chocolate chip cookies to sooth my nerves and worked late into the night fueling myself with carbohydrates) had to give way to something new.

My vision of myself as the "I can have it all" business professional who could push myself to my physical limits with no consequences was shattered. My body had changed, and I knew that my current relationship with my body and the way I treated it on a day-to-day basis was ending.

At first the realization was scary. What was I going to do now? Would I be able to work? I was so accustomed to abusing my body and eating my way through situations that I wasn't sure how I would handle anything in my life.

As I moved through the process, the fear gave way to a sense of relief, and it began to dawn on me that if I faced this condition, lost weight and got my blood sugars under control, I would start to feel better. Taking care of my body, meant taking care of me, and amazingly, once I started doing that, life in general seemed to start taking care of itself.

How to Let Go Of Your "Non-Diabetic" Self

Letting go is incredibly difficult for most people.

In many instances, what holds people back from making a beneficial change is anger at having to make a change in the first place. It could be something as simple as waking up ½ hour early to fit in a morning walk, or choosing not to eat a huge plate of French fries when you go out to lunch on Saturday afternoon.

Whether it's a food or an activity that you want to change, identify the essence of what you enjoyed about it or what need it fulfills. If you can figure out the "essence" of what a food or activity represents to you, then you can find another food or a non-food activity that satisfies you. In some instances you might discover that it was something you don't actually enjoy, but do of habit or because it satisfies an underlying need relating to events or relationships from your past. With some thought you can identify something you can put in its place that will fit the needs of the "new" you.

The exercise below will help you to identify some of the things you enjoyed doing before being diagnosed and how you feel about having to make adjustments as a diabetic (or pre-diabetic).Use this exercise to identify one thing that you enjoy that you know will have to change in order to improve your health. Think about what it means to you and how you feel about making a change. Once you do this, you will be ready to put a new behavior in its place, and you will find you are less resistant to making the change. Use your journal to repeat this exercise whenever you find yourself resistant to making a change that will benefit your health.

Before I was diagnosed with diabetes/pre-diabetes I really enjoyed……..

The thing I like best about (doing this activity/eating this food) is………

Giving up this food/activity or making a change makes me feel………….

A food/activity that I can put in its place is………………..

One of my clients enjoyed going to Starbucks and having a coffee with a "sweet treat" after an evening out with her husband. With the onset of diabetes, she was feeling deprived thinking that she wouldn't be able to do this anymore.

After doing the "letting go" exercise, she discovered that what she really enjoyed was being out with her husband and relaxing after dinner with a good cup of coffee. She liked being in the café, enjoying the atmosphere, which to her seemed a little decadent. Having a sweet was only a part of it. She found that she could still go to Starbucks whenever she wanted if she did a little planning first. This included carrying a very small bottle of natural vanilla syrup in her purse (that she uses to flavor her latte) and bringing her own sugar free treat. A year later she told me "Now that I am not eating those sugar laden, high carb pastries, I feel more in control of my weight and my blood sugar. I'm surprised, but I don't miss them."

Adapting: A Time of Inner Reorientation

The period of adapting is all about moving through the stages of loss and creating a vision for your new beginning. For many people it is an incredibly frustrating time. You are stuck between the old and the new in a place where you know you can't go back, but you don't have a clue how to move forward. Things you might be feeling include anxiety, fear, sadness, or depression.

In their book "You Can't Afford the Luxury of a Negative Thought", John-Roger and Peter McWilliams note that no matter what the loss, the body goes through three phases of recovery. Depending on the type and severity of the loss, the time it takes to go through each stage and the intensity of the feelings at each point along the way will differ. The three stages of recovery include:

❖ Shock/denial

❖ Anger/depression

❖ Understanding/acceptance

It is natural to feel angry, sad, anxious, rebellious and just plain negative when diagnosed with diabetes. You feel all of these emotions because when a loss takes place, the mind, body and emotions go through a process of healing. Feeling lost, sad, angry, or fearful is a natural part of the healing process. The problem arises when you stay stuck in these emotions and are unable to move on to a state of acceptance, where you can take charge of your life and your health in a positive way.

Giving in to the healing process provides us with the ability to adapt to change. One of the biggest mistakes many people make is diving right into action, without also validating their feelings and taking some time for reflection and planning. If they feel angry or depressed, they assume are being "negative", and they are so anxious to immediately accept their loss in a positive light, that they deny the feelings that are a natural part of the change process.

Do take action. But, combine action with taking the time to mourn and to say good-bye to the physical aspects of yourself before your diabetic or pre-diabetic condition. You **will** get to the phase of understanding and acceptance in your own time.

One of the freeing aspects of acceptance is that it gives you the space to let go of a need to see the past in a certain way. This is your opportunity to discover what you really want. At the point of genuine acceptance of your situation, you will find that you have created the space for reflection and for creating the vision of what the new beginning will look like. The exercises in the section "Where Are You Mentally & Spiritually" will help you to set forth a vision of your life as you would like it to unfold.

There are several key things to remember during this time of adapting:

❖ The length and intensity of the healing process differs for every individual.

❖ If you really feel stuck at any point in this phase, seek assistance from your physician or other health care provider.

❖ Following a diagnosis of diabetes or pre-diabetes, it is important to make some initial changes to improve your health, even as you work through the adapting process.

10 Things You Can Do Today

If you have been diagnosed with diabetes or pre-diabetes, and your experience was anything like mine, you probably left your doctor's office with a prescription, a few pamphlets and advice to watch what you eat. Nothing is the same and you are not sure what do about it. Getting control of diabetes will not happen overnight. But, there are a number of things that you can do now that can set you on a path towards controlling your condition and regaining your health.

In his book, "The Art of Getting Well", David Spero, advises, "Make a change, any change at all…even small changes can produce large payoffs. By giving us a sense of control, they set the stage for further growth."

This is a time when you might need to "fake it until you make it." Although you may be feeling scared and unsure what to do, by implementing some initial lifestyle changes that move you towards a better state of health, you will begin to gain the confidence that will set the stage for following through with the new habits and behaviors that you will be learning in The Diabetes Coaching System™.

Try selecting of the suggestions from the list below. Remember, any change is a powerful step towards reaching your goals.

❖ Stop adding sugar to drinks and recipes. There are a number of substitutes, such as Stevia, that you can use if you want to incorporate sweetness in your diet. (Stevia is available in a variety of forms, including a liquid stevia that is offered in a variety of flavors such as Valencia Orange, Dark Chocolate and Lemon Drop)

❖ Add a vegetable to your lunch or dinner. If ever there was a category of foods that can help to improve your health, vegetables are it.

❖ Cut out bread made with grain-based flour. Alternatives include sprouted whole grain bread or breads made with nut, seed, or coconut flour. Even better, forego the bread and try a lettuce wrap.

❖ Lose the white potatoes for a while. If you crave them, substitute a yam or sweet potato that won't have as great an effect on your glucose levels. Or, try some beans with your next meal instead of potatoes. A good source of protein, they are loaded with fiber and are a satisfying alternative to other carbohydrates that affect glucose more dramatically. Cooked white beans with a little olive oil, herbs and a touch of grated cheese are satisfying and delicious.

❖ Add a glass of water to your day. Keeping hydrated helps with your appetite and your overall glucose control. The beverage of choice for everyone, diabetic or not is water. (Note: if your kidney function is compromised or you have congestive heart failure, check with your doctor before increasing your fluid intake) Green tea is another good choice, providing protective antioxidants.

❖ Find a salad dressing you like that does not contain sugar in it. A high quality dressing with olive oil will satisfy you and provide oleic acid (an omega 9 fatty acid that promotes heart health).

❖ Add a handful of nuts to your diet. Nuts contain essential fatty acids that promote cardiovascular health. If you are craving a cookie, add some roasted pumpkin seeds and some sugar free granola to a small portion of nuts for a satisfying snack

❖ Take a walk. It doesn't have to be aerobic. Just getting moving is beneficial. Can't get outside or to the gym? Get some exercise while you watch T.V. Many of us like our television. You don't have to give it up, but why not do a little exercise while you watch? Riding an exercise bike, walking on a treadmill, jumping on a high quality rebound unit or even walking in place are all a step above sitting on the couch. Just 20-30 minutes a day of aerobic exercise daily can be very beneficial. If you have been inactive, check with your doctor before starting

❖ Take a yoga or meditation class. Uncontrolled stress can have an impact on your glucose levels. Stress in your life won't go away, but it's amazing how learning to breathe and to relax can make a difference in how you handle stressful situations. Walking, breathing exercises, hobbies, meditating, yoga, listening to music, and getting enough sleep are all excellent stress busters..

❖ Snack smart. Carry some low fat cheese or vegetables and dip with you to work as a snack so that you have an alternative to the vending machine when that 4pm "gotta have something to eat" feeling hits you. Or, eat a high protein, high fiber bar made with a sugar substitute instead of a piece of candy.

📖 *Reflections:*

As I adapted to my situation, I knew that having a career was still important to me. But, I wanted a life that was more in balance while supporting my well-being and my ability to control my blood sugar levels on a daily basis.

I began to envision a lifestyle where I had more time to spend with my family and time to prepare healthy foods. It included early morning walks in the park with my dog and a home office next to my favorite window where I could gaze out at my favorite trees while I worked. As my vision began to unfold, I knew it would not happen overnight. But with this vision in hand, I was ready and motivated to start a new beginning, not as a victim struggling with an "incurable" illness, but as a woman motivated to improve my lifestyle and empowered to take an active role in controlling my condition.

New Beginnings: Finding Motivation from Within:

There is a fine line that exists between endings, beginnings and the period of adapting. Genuine new beginnings are heralded by a shift in attitude. Along with a renewal of energy, there is a sense of knowing where you want to go, even if you don't yet have a total plan in place for how you will be able to get there.

****

As a practical matter, beginnings are often thrust upon us before we have time to go through the adapting phase.

For example, with diabetes, a beginning of sorts takes place the day of diagnosis. And as mentioned, individuals usually need to start treatment and implement some changes right away. You could think of this as the physical or "external" beginning.

But, at the point of diagnosis, our mind and emotions have not yet caught up with the physical change that is now manifesting itself. So, in many instances we find ourselves playing catch up with our mind and spirit while attending to physical or external needs on a day-to-day basis.

How do you know when you are truly embarking on a new beginning?

Embarking on a new beginning does not mean that you will never feel sad, depressed or angry. It doesn't mean you have all the answers.

The hallmark of embarking upon a new beginning is that you are no longer motivated by a set of external "shoulds" thrust upon you by doctors, health care practitioners or well-meaning friends and relatives. Instead your motivation comes from within, driven by your hopes, dreams, and vision of your future.

With a renewed sense of purpose, you are ready to move forward.

Action Steps

❖ If you find yourself stuck and unable to move forward with your diabetes program, ask yourself these questions and record your observations and feelings in your journal. What has ended for me? How do I feel about it? (you may want to go back to the "letting go" exercise to help you identify what is holding you back)

❖ Find a support person that you can talk to and brainstorm with in order to get clear about what is holding you back and how you might be able to address your feelings.

❖ Examine some of the major changes/transition periods in your life. How did you react then? When change comes do you tend to ignore, deny or embrace endings?

❖ If you are ready to move forward, how does it feel? Exciting? A little scary? What do you want to accomplish?

THE LIVE FREE BLOOD SUGAR & DIABETES COACHING SYSTEM™

As discussed in the first section of the workbook, the LIVE FREE Blood Sugar & Diabetes Coaching System™ is an outgrowth of my experiences both as a change management consultant and recovering diabetic. It has a strong foundation in coaching concepts designed to provide structure and motivation throughout the lifestyle change process.

I organized the program into a series of steps in order to clarify the various elements of the process. Change, however, is not a linear process. You may find yourself working on one or more steps at any given time. The important thing is to understand how all of the steps come together to enable you to be successful in managing your blood sugars and overall health. Although this is not a "phased program", you will note that the first letters in each of the steps form two distinct acronyms: LIVE and FREE.

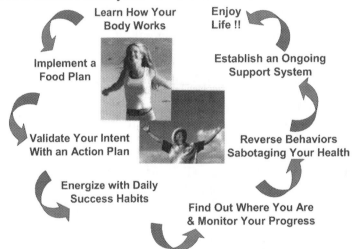

LIVE: The first steps in the coaching system are designed to empower you to change your daily habits, particularly when obstacles get in your way. You will learn how to balance your blood sugars and how to stay on track and motivated in the face of life's daily challenges. These steps include:

- ❖ Learn How Your Body Works
- ❖ Implement a Food Plan
- ❖ Validate Your Intent with an Action Plan
- ❖ Energize with Daily Success Habits

FREE: Once you have begun to implement new lifestyle habits, it becomes important to totally free yourself from old behaviors so that you can continue to move forward. The final four steps in the coaching system encompass this process. These steps include:

- ❖ Find out Where You Are and Monitor Your Progress
- ❖ Reverse Behaviors Sabotaging Your Health
- ❖ Establish an Ongoing Support Team
- ❖ Enjoy Life

The infomation below provides a brief explanation of each step in the LIVE FREE Blood Sugar & Diabetes Coaching System™. The remaining sections of the book will lead you through each step, providing guidance and support as you begin to implement your plan and new lifestyle habits.

Learn How Your Body Works

You do not have to be a medical expert to develop a stronger connection to your body and to learn how to live in harmony with the way your body works. But, in order to control blood sugar levels, it is critical that you are aware of all of your options and have the basic knowledge needed to make informed decisions about your health.

Implement a Food Plan

Implementing a food plan with a focus on eating nutrient dense foods will support a healthy, balanced physical state that will enable your body mechanisms to function properly. Although there are many components to conquering diabetes, what you eat on a daily basis is going to have a major impact on keeping your blood sugars under control.

Validate Your Intent with an Action Plan

Goals plus an action plan provide much needed direction and a means of measuring progress. Your action plan will keep you focused so that you can achieve your desired results.

Energize with Success Habits

A plan is meaningless without consistent daily actions that lead you forward. Success habits in the areas of eating, exercise, and stress management will support your ability to give your pancreas a much needed rest from the onslaught of refined foods and chronic stress that wreak havoc with your ability to maintain a healthy weight, increase your energy levels, and keep your blood sugars under control.

Find Out Where You Are & Monitor Your Progress

Whenever you are adopting new patterns of behavior, there will be times when life's challenges get in the way. Monitoring your progress by testing your blood sugars on a daily basis, keeping a daily journal and making periodic assessments of your progress will help you to stay on track and to make necessary adjustments in your daily routine.

Reverse Behaviors Sabotaging Your Health

When trying to conquer a chronic condition, one of the most important things you can do is to learn how to eliminate behaviors that sabotage your efforts. Managing your mind, including making peace with your relationship with food, is truly one of the secrets to vibrant health.

Establish an Ongoing Support System

It is impossible to conquer a chronic health condition on your own. Building a support team and staying connected to people that can assist you is another key strategy for managing blood sugars and making lasting lifestyle changes.

Enjoy Life

Healthy living is important for managing diabetes, but it is not the end goal. Enjoying the gift of life and experiencing your life's purpose is the ultimate gift of vibrant health. So, live each day to the fullest. Learn how to conquer worry, manage stress, and remember to have fun.

❶ Learn How Your Body Works

Information is Empowerment

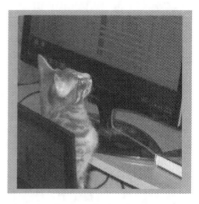

When it comes to making lifestyle changes, having an understanding of how and why you should make those changes will increase your ability to make changes that will last. I believe that the learning process is so critical to your success that my entire program is based upon teaching you what you need to know about your body, food and exercise so that you no longer have to be dependent upon "diet" experts for the latest fad. You won't have to count, measure or feel deprived because you are going to learn how to eat and live in harmony with the way your body was designed to work.

Every choice you make will take you either towards or away from the vision of health you desire for yourself. If you gain knowledge about the physical aspects of diabetes, you will have a better understanding of how your choices affect your body's ability to function properly, and you will gain more confidence in making choices that lead you towards a healthier state of being.

You don't need to become a medical expert to gain a basic understanding of the relationship between diabetes and how your body functions. But, if you want to be proactive in making informed decisions about own health and lifestyle, you will need to have both a general understanding of what is going on inside your body and information about the options available to you.

Gaining information about diabetes and healthy living will empower you to:

❖ Make the connection between your physical condition and the behaviors that affect your physical health

❖ Work effectively with your medical providers,

❖ Make informed decisions, and

❖ Take action to achieve your lifestyle goals.

The Diabetes Primer

If you have diabetes, pre-diabetes, or risk factors, every day you will need to make lifestyle choices, including what to eat, how much to exercise, and whether to take supplements. Although experts agree on many healthy living concepts, there are just as many areas where the experts disagree, particularly when it comes to what you should or shouldn't eat for blood sugar control. So in the end, the choices are yours to make.

You do not need to learn everything there is to know about how your pancreas works or about nutrition. But, understanding the basic physical nature of diabetes coupled with gaining knowledge about diet, exercise and stress management will enable you to develop the confidence to make informed decisions about how to manage your condition.

Food, Energy and Diabetes

❖ Cells need energy, and the fuel of choice for cells is the simple sugar glucose.

❖ Carbohydrates are the primary food source for glucose.

❖ The digestive system processes carbohydrates, breaking them down into glucose, so that the carbohydrates are converted into a form that is usable by our cells.

❖ Insulin transports glucose to cells and regulates the balance of glucose in the body.

❖ When the body's digestive and related self-regulating mechanisms break down anywhere in the process, diabetes and other chronic conditions result.

The process of taking in food and transforming that food into life sustaining energy is one of the most important aspects of a person's health. Think of your body as a huge chemical processing plant. Through the food we eat, chemicals are taken in, processed by various types of reactions and then distributed throughout the body to be used immediately or stored.

❖ The foods we eat can be grouped into three major categories: carbohydrates, proteins and fats. In reality, most foods are a combination of these nutrients, i.e. proteins generally contain fat and carbohydrate foods frequently contain some fat and protein. The only foods that are virtually 100% fat are oils, butter and margarine.

❖ When our digestion process is working properly, carbohydrates from the foods we eat are broken down into their basic elements: short chain molecules including glucose, fructose and galactose, which are then absorbed from the small intestine into the blood stream where they are available as a source of energy to the cells.

❖ When delivered to the body's blood circulation, the absorbed carbohydrates cause an elevation of the blood glucose concentration. The body responds by releasing insulin into the blood. Insulin's job is to clear sugar from the blood by facilitating the distribution of the glucose to the muscle cells for fuel and to the liver and fat cells for storage.

❖ A portion of glucose remains in the blood to serve the proper functioning of the brain and central nervous system. (The normal level is approximately 80 to 100 mg/dl.)

Over time, the pattern of the extent and duration of the blood glucose rise that occurs after you eat has a profound effect upon your body's ability to regulate the amount of glucose that remains in your blood. As we will learn in the following pages, when we eat foods that are digested more slowly, the insulin response is moderated, our cells are nourished, we feel energized and we experience a sense of well-being. But, when we eat an overabundance of foods that cause fast rises in glucose accompanied by a sharp rise in insulin,(such as sugar and refined carbohydrates) the body loses its ability to self-regulate, the process breaks down, and diabetes and other chronic illnesses can result.

The relationship between the digestive process and the metabolism of carbohydrates is described on the following pages

Digestion: Turning Food into Energy

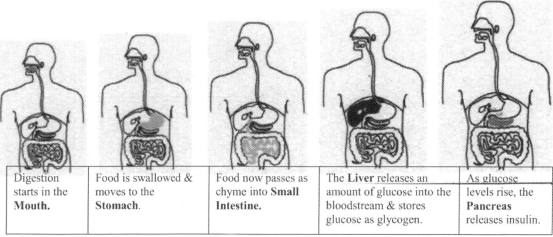

Digestion starts in the **Mouth.**	Food is swallowed & moves to the **Stomach**.	Food now passes as chyme into **Small Intestine.**	The **Liver** releases an amount of glucose into the bloodstream & stores glucose as glycogen.	As glucose levels rise, the **Pancreas** releases insulin.

CHEWING: The digestion process begins the minute we take food into our mouths. Here the food is broken down into smaller particles by chewing.

❖ The food is mixed with the salivary enzymes that begin the process of digestion. The saliva breaks down starches into dextrin and maltose. #

SWALLOWING: After we chew our food, it is swallowed and pushed through the esophagus to the stomach.

PROCESSING: After the food has been processed by the muscular and chemical actions of the stomach, the *chyme* (which is what your food is now called) passes into the first part of the small intestine.

❖ In the small intestine, the chyme is mixed with the enzymes from the pancreas and bile from the liver/gallbladder. These enzymes further the process of digestion by breaking down proteins into amino acids, the carbohydrates and sugars into glucose, and the fats into fatty acids.

DELIVERY: In the next phase of the small intestine, the components of the food are absorbed and actively transported through the intestinal walls into the blood stream where they are available as a source of energy to the cells.

❖ Glucose (from carbohydrates) is absorbed from the intestines into the blood where it travels to the liver and other organs.

❖ The liver is programmed to release a certain amount of glucose into the blood and to store a portion for later use. (it is stored as "glycogen")

❖ When delivered to the body's blood circulation, the absorbed carbohydrates cause an elevation of the blood glucose concentration.

❖ In response to the rising level of glucose, the pancreas is triggered to secrete insulin into the bloodstream and to transport the glucose into cells where it can be used for energy.

As you will learn on the following pages, maintaining an amount of glucose in the bloodstream to promote optimal health is a delicate balancing act. In the next section we will explore how the liver and pancreas work together to keep your blood sugar levels steady.

The Pancreas, Liver, and Insulin Connection

In order to protect the proper functioning of your brain and nervous system, you must maintain a fairly constant level of blood glucose. As you have learned, glucose is produced as a result of the digestion of carbohydrates from the food that we eat.

But you aren't eating all the time. You go without food between meals, sometimes you skip meals and of course you aren't eating while you sleep. Regardless of when or how much you eat, your body tries to maintain a consistent supply of glucose for your cells by maintaining a constant level of glucose in your bloodstream.

Without the ability to regulate the amount of glucose in your blood, your cells would have more than enough glucose right after a meal and starve in between meals and overnight. Additionally, too much glucose remaining in the bloodstream can have damaging effects throughout your body.

Hormones That Regulate Blood Sugar Levels

The pancreas is a large gland that is located in the abdomen, behind your stomach. The main function of the pancreas is to produce insulin, digestive enzymes, and other hormones. To maintain the proper balance of glucose in your blood, the pancreas produces two hormones: insulin and glycogen.

These hormones are produced by different types of cells in the pancreas and have opposite actions which together regulate the (glucose) levels in your body.

INSULIN:	GLUCAGON:
Is produced by the BETA cells of pancreas	Is produced by the ALPHA cells of the pancreas
Is released when you have just eaten, and the level of glucose in your bloodstream is high.	Is released when your blood sugar levels are low (for example, if you have been fasting or exercising)
Stimulates the cells within your body to take up the glucose in your blood and to use the glucose either for immediate energy or for storing (as glycogen, a starchy substance stored both in the liver and muscle cells).	Stimulates the liver and muscles to break down stored glycogen and release the glucose into the bloodstream so that it can be used for energy.
When you have an oversupply of glucose, your body stores the excess in the liver and muscles as glycogen, or if there is too much glucose, it stores it as fat.	When glucose is in short supply, your body mobilizes glucose from stored glycogen and/or stimulates you to eat food.

The action of insulin prevents the blood glucose concentration (as well as the concentrations of fatty acids and amino acids) from substantially increasing in the bloodstream. In this way, your body maintains a steady blood glucose concentration.

Maintaining the Balance of Insulin and Glucagon

How does your body know when to secrete glucagon or insulin? If your body is functioning normally, the levels of insulin and glucagon are counter-balanced in the bloodstream in the following way:

High Glucose Levels ⟹ Beta Cells Produce Insulin

⬇

Glucose is Absorbed into Cells ⟹ Utilized as Energy or Stored as Glycogen

❖ After you eat, digest, and absorb carbohydrate foods, your blood glucose level rises and your body prepares to receive the glucose, fatty acids and amino acids that have been absorbed from the food.

❖ The presence of these substances in the intestine stimulates the pancreatic beta cells to release insulin into the blood. (and also inhibits the pancreatic alpha cells from secreting glucagon)

❖ The levels of insulin in the blood begin to rise, and the release of insulin into the bloodstream facilitates the ability of cells (particularly liver, fat and muscle) to absorb the incoming molecules of glucose, fatty acids, and amino acids.

❖ Insulin acts as a "key", essentially unlocking tiny doors on cell walls (called insulin receptor sites) that allow glucose to enter the cells.

❖ As part of this process, insulin activates the production of glucose transporters within the cells. These specialized protein molecules emerge from the nuclei of the cells to grab glucose from the blood and bring it to the interiors of the cells. Once inside the cell, glucose can be utilized as an immediate power source to provide fuel for energy-requiring functions.

❖ If there is more glucose than is immediately needed for energy, insulin stimulates the liver and muscle cells to store the glucose in the form of glycogen for use when it is needed at a later time. If there is too much glucose on a regular basis, it will be stored as fat.

Low Glucose Levels ⟹ Alpha Cells Produce Glucagon

⬇

Glucagon "Instructs Liver and Muscle to Convert Glycogen into Glucose

❖ In contrast, when you are between meals or sleeping, your body is essentially starving. Your cells need supplies of glucose from the blood in order to keep going.

❖ During these times, slight drops in blood sugar levels stimulate glucagon secretion from the pancreatic alpha cells and inhibit insulin secretion from the beta cells.

❖ As blood-glucagon levels rise, glucagon acts on liver, muscle and kidney tissue to initiate a process to make glucose that gets released into the blood. In simple terms the glucagon "instructs" the liver and muscles to begin converting glycogen to glucose. This action prevents the blood-glucose concentration from falling drastically.

Insulin Resistance and Type 2 Diabetes

The life promoting qualities of insulin can be a double edge sword when there is too much glucose or too much insulin in the bloodstream on a habitual basis. Few people realize that once glycogen storage sites in the muscles and liver are filled, excess glucose remaining in the bloodstream is converted to and stored as fat. This is just one of the consequences of habitual high blood sugar levels.

🔑 Our bodies were not designed to handle an onslaught of refined foods and sugar on a daily basis. As you will learn in the following pages, the result of habitually eating highly processed and refined foods coupled with weight gain and a sedentary lifestyle is for many the path to a condition known as insulin resistance.

When people are insulin resistant, their muscle, fat, and liver cells do not respond properly to insulin. As a result, their bodies need more insulin to help glucose enter cells. The pancreas tries to keep up with this increased demand for insulin by producing more. Eventually, the pancreas fails to keep up with the body's need for insulin. Excess glucose builds up in the bloodstream, setting the stage for diabetes. Many people with insulin resistance have high levels of both glucose and insulin circulating in their blood at the same time

❖ On the surface it seems that having excess insulin is a good thing. You might think that if we have more insulin than we need, we will always have enough to keep our blood sugar under control, and hence we won't get diabetes or have other problems. But, it is just the opposite.

❖ Too much insulin causes a whole host of problems, including the development of hypoglycemia and weight gain. Insulin resistance is often a precursor to Type 2 diabetes, particularly if left uncontrolled.

Below is a more detailed description of what occurs regarding the interaction of insulin with cells when insulin resistance is present:

❖ The pancreas produces and releases insulin into the bloodstream in response to an increase in blood glucose.

❖ Insulin interacts with the surface of cells, but has difficulty opening the passageway, which subsequently prevents sufficient glucose from entering the cells.

❖ Since the glucose cannot enter the cells, it remains in the bloodstream.

❖ The pancreas responds by producing and releasing more insulin into the bloodstream.

❖ Blood glucagon levels rise, and glucagon acts on the liver, muscle, and kidney tissue, "instructing" these tissues to begin converting glycogen to glucose.

❖ The end result is that excess glucose gets released into the blood, and insulin takes the extra glucose and transports it into fat storage.

On the following pages we will explore what happens when the system breaks down and the body can no longer maintain the delicate balancing act that keeps our blood sugars in a normal range.

Insulin and Fat Storage

As the preceding sections demonstrate, there is a complex relationship between food, blood sugar, insulin, and fat.

☛ Few people realize that in addition to helping to regulate blood sugar levels, insulin also helps to store fat. Yes, insulin is a powerful fat-building hormone.

You have learned that after you eat, digest, and absorb carbohydrate foods, your blood sugar level normally rises. Then the pancreas responds by releasing insulin, which transports the glucose into your cells where it can be used as energy.

Most people are surprised to learn that insulin has anything to do with fat storage. But, now you know that when you have more glucose in your body than your cells need, insulin takes the extra glucose and transports it into fat storage. Then, blood sugar levels return to normal. This is in one sense a good thing, because it helps (at least in the short term) to prevent high levels of glucose remaining in the bloodstream. But, when insulin levels rise and spike in an effort to control high blood sugar levels, more fat is also being stored.

Visceral Obesity and Insulin Resistance:

Having high insulin levels on a consistent basis means more body fat. Another important concept to be aware of is that not all body fat is the same, and when it comes to diabetes, of particular concern is a type of body fat often referred to as "visceral obesity."

☛ Visceral obesity is a type of obesity in which fat is concentrated around the middle of the body, particularly surrounding the intestines. Visceral fat is linked to extra fat storage in the liver (which can raise blood sugar levels) and to extra fat in muscle cells, making them resistant to insulin.

****

Without regular physical activity, which burns glucose and lowers insulin levels, insulin keeps increasing the ratio of fat cells to muscle cells. With more fat cells and fewer muscle cells, the body loses still more of its ability to efficiently burn up glucose, and ultimately, both glucose and insulin levels remain elevated.

Visceral obesity is evident when you have a waist measurement greater than the circumference of your hips. In most cases, individuals with visceral obesity have some degree of insulin resistance. This problem is made worse by the fact that the more overweight you are, the more resistant to insulin you tend to become.

One reason this happens is because extra adipose tissue ("fat") produces a hormone called resistin, which makes it harder for insulin to escort sugar into the cells. Subsequently, too much fat results in the production of even more resistin.

In the following section, we will see review how the cycle of insulin resistance builds and can lead to diabetes.

The Vicious Cycle of Insulin Resistance

❖ When your body is not responding fully to insulin, your cells absorb less glucose from your bloodstream, which causes you to have high blood glucose levels. This results in less glucose being utilized by your cells.

❖ When your cells are not absorbing enough glucose, your mind and body perceive that the body is starving.

❖ Your pancreatic alpha cells react by secreting more glucagon, and the glucagon levels in your blood rise.

❖ Glucagon then acts on your liver and muscles to breakdown stored glycogen and to release even more glucose into the blood, further raising your blood-glucose levels.

❖ The pancreas reacts by producing more insulin. This in turn, as we have learned, leads to more fat. It's a vicious cycle. As the body tries to compensate, glucose and insulin levels swing from high to low and back again. Over years, the weight gain increases and the pancreas begins to exhaust itself.

As the situation worsens your burnt out pancreas is producing less insulin while struggling to keep up with ever increasing blood glucose levels.

You might be wondering why the body's ability to store excess glucose in the muscles and liver as glycogen, does not spare us from having high levels of glucose floating in our bloodstream. The problem is that the ability of our cells to store glycogen is not infinite. If glycogen starts to build up to high levels in the liver, the liver will repress additional synthesis. As a result, when more glucose continues to enter the liver cells, it is redirected into a different metabolic pathway.

With some simplification, here is what happens: Within this metabolic pathway, fatty acids are made and then transported out of the liver as *lipoproteins*. While circulating, these lipoproteins are broken apart into free-floating fatty acids that are utilized by other tissues. Certain tissues in our body then use the fatty acids in order to make triglycerides.

Repeated high blood glucose sets the stage for an imbalanced state whereby:

❖ Fats in the blood feeding the liver cause insulin resistance

❖ Insulin resistance causes elevated blood sugar and insulin levels

❖ Elevated insulin levels cause the fat cells to build even more abdominal fat

❖ This process raises triglycerides in the liver's blood supply, which in turn causes blood sugar and insulin levels to increase because of increased resistance to insulin.

❖ Ultimately, a vicious cycle is created until either the imbalance leads to full blown diabetes or lifestyle changes are made that can restore the body to a state of health.

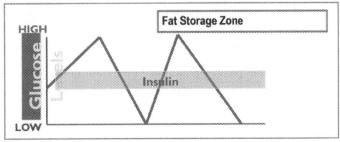

Insulin Resistance and Hypoglycemia:

If you have insulin resistance and constantly eat foods such as refined carbohydrates, a lot more insulin is needed to bring your blood sugar back down to healthy levels. Some people with insulin resistance produce so much insulin that their blood sugar levels dive way below normal, causing a condition called hypoglycemia. Hypoglycemia causes uncomfortable reactions such as jitteriness, tiredness, mental dullness, headaches, or intense cravings for sugary or starchy foods. Even though the hallmark of hypoglycemia is low blood sugar, and diabetes is characterized by high blood sugar, the root cause, i.e. the inability to process carbohydrates effectively is the same. Many people who experience ongoing hypoglycemia later end up with Type 2 diabetes.

Why Weight Loss is Important

- ❖ Experts note that even modest weight loss helps overcome insulin resistance and bring blood sugar levels down. In fact, many Type 2 diabetics find that the combination of losing weight and modest exercise enables them to reduce or eliminate their medications.

- ❖ Studies have shown that you can significantly lower your risk of getting full flown diabetes by losing as little as 5-10% of your body weight and exercising as little as ½ hour per day.

Reaching and maintaining a reasonable weight is an important component of your overall plan to improve your health.

How does weight loss help you to control your blood glucose levels?

- ❖ When you lose weight, cells become more sensitive to insulin so that the body uses insulin more effectively.

- ❖ The result of more effective use of insulin is that insulin is able to move more glucose from the bloodstream into your cells.

- ❖ Your cells are now able to use needed glucose for energy.

- ❖ The end result is an improvement in blood glucose levels, which for many diabetics means the ability to lower the dosage of glucose-lowering pills or in some instances eliminating medication or insulin injections.

If your weight is not within the guidelines for your height and age, (check with your physician) start thinking about weight loss as a key goal for your overall plan.

In final section of the Diabetes Primer you will learn the role that sugar, refined and highly processed carbohydrates play in fostering the rise of diabetes and why a nation eating low fat sugary cookies, snacks and other processed foods is getting fatter and fatter. The good news is that as you lose body fat, insulin resistance improves too. This is why in a later section "Reverse Situations Negatively Affecting Your Health", the importance of losing weight is emphasized as an initial step towards avoiding or managing diabetes.

Diabetes: The Body in Crisis

From the above discussion three things are evident:

❖ First, our cells need energy in the form of glucose,

❖ Second, the glucose has to be delivered to and absorbed by our cells for it to do any good, and

❖ Third, there is a delicate balance of insulin and blood sugar that needs to be maintained in order for our bodies to function properly.

When the body's digestive and related self-regulating mechanisms break down anywhere in the process, diabetes and other chronic conditions result. Diabetes is a disease in which the body does not produce or properly use insulin, a hormone that is needed to convert glucose into the energy needed for daily life.

TYPE 1 DIABETES: the pancreas either no longer produces insulin or it doesn't produce enough of it.

TYPE 2 DIABETES: your pancreas makes insulin, but you experience high glucose levels either because

1) The pancreas may not be producing insulin in sufficient quantity,

2) The body's cells may have lost their ability to respond to insulin - even if the pancreas is producing enough insulin, or

3) A combination of these two factors.

The two major forms of diabetes have different causes, although both are characterized by elevated blood sugars and insulin problems.

The treatment for Type 1 and Type 2 diabetes is also different, primarily because Type 1 is characterized by an inability of the pancreas to produce insulin, so that treatment always includes the replacement of insulin via injections or pump (in addition to patches and sprays currently being developed).

Treatment options for Type 2 diabetes may range from adjusting diet and exercise to taking oral medications, or in some cases insulin is required.

Even though treatment may differ, making lifestyle changes are critical for both Type 1 and Type 2 diabetics. It is true that Type 1 diabetics will always need to replace insulin, but with a good program of diet, exercise and nutritional support, Type 1 diabetics will be able to more effectively manage their insulin use and avoid complications.

Pre-Diabetes and the Progression to Type 2 Diabetes

Pre-diabetes is a condition where an individual has levels of sugar in the bloodstream that are higher than normal, but not yet high enough to be classified as diabetes. Pre-diabetes can be detected with a number of different blood tests.

❖ **HBA1C SCREENING TEST**: A blood test that measures the level of Hemoglobin A1C in your blood to indicate your average blood glucose over a 2-3 month period.

- ❖ **Fasting Plasma Glucose**: After an 8 to 12 hour fast, your blood is drawn and blood sugar levels measured. A reading of less than 100 mg/dl is normal; 100 to 125 indicates pre-diabetes and 126 or higher is a sign of full blown diabetes.

- ❖ **Oral Glucose Tolerance Test:** the OGTT measures blood glucose after a person fasts for at least 8 hours and 2 hours after the person drinks a liquid containing 75 grams of glucose dissolved in water. It tells the doctor how your body processes glucose

The chart below shows the progression that often begins with insulin resistance, leading to pre-diabetes that, without intervention, can develop into full blown Type 2 diabetes.

Type 2 Diabetes Progression

A1C

Fasting Plasma Glucose Test (FPG)

Oral Glucose Tolerance Test (OGTT)

DIABETES

Disorder in body's means of utilizing Glucose

- • A1C 6.5 or above
- • FGP 126 or above
- • OGTT 200 or above

"PRE-DIABETES"

An early form of diabetes (sometimes referred to as Impaired Fasting Glucose or Impaired Glucose Tolerance), depending upon the test used for diagnosis. Pre-diabetes frequently leads to a full blown form of the disease and can slowly cause many of the same complications if not brought under control.

- • A1C 5.7-6.4
- • FGP 100-125
- • OGTT 140-199

INSULIN RESISTANCE

A condition whereby there is a decrease in the ability of the body's cells to respond to insulin. In this case, more insulin than usual is required to keep blood sugar levels under control.

Often without symptoms & test results may be normal.

The Problem with Excess Glucose

When levels of glucose in the bloodstream get too high, blood cells can begin to cease to circulate as freely as they should. In effect, the blood of a diabetic becomes too "sticky". As a result, certain tissue can become seriously deprived of vital nutrients and oxygen. Damaging effects of excess glucose in the bloodstream include:

❖ **Cellular accumulation of sorbitol, a by-product of glucose metabolism**. High concentrations of glucose can lead to the cellular accumulation of sorbitol. The buildup of sorbitol within cells causes them to swell and damage tissue. This can lead to complications of eyes and nerves.

❖ **Glycation**. This is a process by which glucose binds to, chemically alters, and damages proteins. This process results in the formation of advanced glycation end products referred to as "AGEs." AGEs form at a constant but slow rate in the normal body. Their formation, however, is markedly accelerated in uncontrolled diabetes because of the increased availability of glucose. Over time these altered proteins may accumulate in the cells and interfere with their normal functions. Complications of the eyes, kidneys and circulatory system are associated with these altered proteins.

❖ **Increased production of free radicals.** Elevated levels of glucose increase the production of free radicals. Although free radicals are a natural by-product of normal cellular metabolism, free radical damage has been linked to heart disease, cancer and other degenerative disorders.

Possible Diabetic Complications

The goal of any type of diabetes care is to keep blood sugar levels as normal as possible. As the following statistics from the American Diabetes Association show, uncontrolled diabetes can take an enormous toll.

❖ **Blindness**: The number one cause of blindness in people age 2 to 70 is diabetic retinopathy. Every year up to 24,000 Americans lose their sight because of vascular complications caused by diabetes. Glaucoma and cataracts are also more common in individuals with diabetes.

❖ **Kidney Failure**: Diabetes is the leading cause of kidney failure and is responsible for 40% of all new cases. At least 100,000 diabetics are currently undergoing dialysis or have received kidney transplants.

❖ **Nerve Damage**: Diabetic neuropathy affects 60 to 70 percent of all diabetics. Symptoms range from mild loss of sensation in the feet to constant pain in various parts of the body. Nerve damage may also impair digestion and cause other complications.

❖ **Amputations:** More than 56,000 amputations are performed every year on patients with diabetes, making this condition the leading cause of non-traumatic amputations.

❖ **Cardiovascular disease:** Elevated blood sugar damages the blood vessels and alters blood lipid levels. High triglyceride levels are common in diabetics, as are low levels of protective HDL cholesterol. In addition, hypertension affects almost 60% of individuals with Type 2 diabetes. People who have diabetes are two to four times more likely to develop heart disease or have a stroke than non-diabetics and three-fourths of all diabetics (more than 77,000 annually) ultimately die of heart disease.

Know the Risk Factors and Symptoms of Diabetes

If you are concerned about developing diabetes, but have not been diagnosed, the following information about risk factors and symptoms will assist you to determine if testing is warranted.

RISK FACTORS: If you have any of the following risk factors, you may be at an increased risk for diabetes. You should be particularly vigilant for the symptoms of diabetes and getting tested. Discuss any concerns you have with your physician.

- Family History
- 20% over a healthy weight or obese
- Sedentary Lifestyle
- You are African-American, Latino, Asian, Native American or Pacific Islander
- Diabetes during pregnancy or had a baby who was 9 lb. or more at birth
- Low HDL (good cholesterol) or high overall cholesterol levels
- Very high blood pressure or very high triglycerides

SYMPTOMS OF DIABETES: Diabetes has a number of symptoms that you might not suspect are associated with the disease. If you have one or more of these symptoms, discuss diabetes testing with your physician.

- Frequent urination
- Excessive thirst
- Unexplained weight loss
- Unusual hunger
- Extreme fatigue
- Irritability
- Frequent infections
- Blurred vision
- Slow to heal cuts & bruises
- Vaginitis or recurring yeast infections in women
- Tingling or numbness in hands or feet
- Recurring skin, gum or bladder infections

SYMPTOMS OF INSULIN RESISTANCE: Below is a list of some of the most common symptoms of insulin resistance, a pre-cursor to diabetes. It is very possible to affect the progression of diabetes by making lifestyle changes. If you are experiencing one or more of these symptoms, speak with your physician, especially if you have risk factors for diabetes.

- ❖ **Fatigue**. The failure of insulin to work properly and the inability of your cells to get sufficient glucose eventually take its toll on the body. Some people with insulin resistance are tired in the morning or afternoon, others are exhausted all day.

- ❖ **Low blood sugar**. Prolonged periods of hypoglycemia, accompanied by many of the symptoms listed here, especially physical and mental fatigue, may be symptoms of insulin resistance.

- ❖ **Sleepiness**. Many people with insulin resistance get sleepy immediately after eating a meal containing more than 20% or 30% carbohydrates. This is often a pasta meal, or even a meat meal that includes potatoes or bread and a sweet dessert.

- ❖ **Increased weight and fat storage**. In males, a large abdomen is the more obvious and earliest sign of insulin resistance. In females, it can be a large abdomen and/or prominent buttocks.

- ❖ **Increased triglycerides**. Individuals typically may have stores of excess triglycerides in their arteries as a result of insulin resistance.

Take Time to Assess Your Physical Condition

Before you start any program it is a good idea to get a handle on where you are physically for a variety of reasons. Most importantly, you want to make sure that any decisions you make will not exacerbate any underlying conditions that you may not be aware of and that you are aligning your action plan with your physical state and unique biochemistry. The following section sets forth some suggestions for assessing your physical condition followed by an explanation of the key tests that you should be aware of.

- **Get A Physical**: Have you had a yearly physical that includes basic testing? Do you know your fasting glucose level? Lipid profile?

- **Take a Health Assessment**: Review your health history and concerns with a coach or other health practitioner to identify areas where you would like to implement changes so that you can work together to reach your goals.

- **Know Your Risk Factors for Heart Disease**: In addition to other tests used to assess heart problems, speak with your physician about having your Homocysteine and C-Reactive Protein levels tested. Another non-invasive procedure known as Intima Media Thickness scanning (IMT) is a safe and relatively inexpensive means of predicting the risk of heath attack or stroke.

- **Determine Your Risk For Diabetes:** Do you know your family history? If you have risk factors or symptoms, consult your physician to discuss testing.

- **If Diabetic, Know Your Numbers:** Do you test your blood sugars regularly? Do you know your average blood sugar levels based on an HBA1C test**?**

- **Check Your Weight:** Is it within the range for your height and age? Do you know your muscle mass to fat ratio? What is your waist circumference?

- **Check Your Blood Pressure:** Is it within the normal range? If you don't know, make arrangements to have your blood pressure tested. If it is not within normal range, discuss treatment with your physician.

- **Check Your Exercise & Fitness Level:** Do you get some form of exercise at least once a day? If you don't currently have an exercise program, confirm that you don't have any conditions that would impede starting an exercise routine.

- **Review Your Medications:** Regarding any medications you may be taking, do you know the type, long term effects, contraindications, alternatives, and the overall course of action recommended by your physician? If you have any questions or concerns, review them with your doctor.

- **Take Care of Your Eyes and Feet:** If diabetic, have you had your eyes and feet examined at least yearly? If not schedule an appointment.

- **Take Care of Your Kidneys:** If diabetic, have you had your microalbumin levels measured? If not, discuss having this test performed with your physician.

- **If Symptomatic, Check for Thyroid Disease:** If you have any symptoms of thyroid disease, have you scheduled a TSH test? If the results were within normal range, have you discussed more in-depth testing with your physician in order to test the levels of the T_4 and T_3 thyroid hormones in your blood? Speak with your family physician or a specialist if your TSH test is within normal range but your symptoms persist.

Tests to Be Aware Of

When it comes to your health, what you don't know can hurt you. For example, uncontrolled diabetes or undiagnosed heart conditions can lead to serious complications. The following section sets forth a few of the key tests that you should be aware of.

"LIPID PROFILE" (TOTAL CHOLESTEROL, HDL, LDL, TRIGLYCERIDES)

	What is it?	ADA recommendations for people with Diabetes
Total Cholesterol	Cholesterol is a waxy substance produced by the liver or supplied in the diet, through animal products such as meat, poultry, fish and dairy products. Cholesterol does not dissolve in the blood, so it must be carried through the bloodstream by proteins, called lipoproteins. The most common cause for elevation in total cholesterol is the combination of sugar, starch and saturated fat in the diet, which increases "bad" cholesterol"	Total cholesterol should be less than 200 mg/dL.
Low Density Lipoprotein (LDL)	LDL carries cholesterol through the blood and is often called the "bad" cholesterol. When there is too much LDL cholesterol in the blood, it combines with other substances to form deposits on the blood vessel walls. This causes a narrowing of the blood vessels and increases the risk of heart attack.	LDL should be less than 100 mg/dL
High Density Lipoprotein (HDL)	Often called the "good" cholesterol, HDL removes cholesterol from the blood vessel walls and carries it back to the liver to be disposed of. HDL cholesterol can be raised by regular exercise or weight loss. It can also be improved by consuming a daily diet low in sugar starch and trans fat.	HDL should be greater than 4o mg/dL (Men) or greater than 55 mg/dL (Women).
Triglycerides	Triglycerides are a combination of three fatty acids found in the foods we eat. Insulin allows triglycerides to enter the fat cells for storage. If this process does not take place properly and the triglycerides stay in the bloodstream, this can lead to heart disease. Maintaining a diet low in sugar, starch and saturated fats will help to keep triglyceride levels in check. Note that the higher your triglycerides, the lower your good cholesterol levels will be.	Triglycerides goals should be less than 150

 Cholesterol levels are just one piece of the heart health equation.

Cholesterol is fatty oil that can't travel around in your bloodstream on its own. It needs to be packed into what are known as "particles. And the number and size of these particles matter when it comes to heart health. The particles are what deliver the bad cholesterol inside the walls of the artery to form plaque, and the more particles you have, the greater your risk for heart disease. This number is known as LDL-P, and you want this number to be less than 700. And small dense particles are more likely to damage our artery wall as they can enter more easily than larger LDL particles. So you also want to include testing for levels of sdLDL to understand if you have a large number of small dense LDL particles.

Another type of cholesterol you might want to be aware of, especially if you have diabetes or pre-diabetes, is Lp(a) cholesterol. With an attached "corkscrew" called apoprotein (a), Lp(a) is an inherited trait that can increase risk of heart disease and stroke. Having high levels of this form of LDL, can be un-nerving because there is very little that can be done in terms of lifestyle to bring Lp(a) down. But, the good news is that being even more vigilant with of your other lipid numbers can help with your overall risk for heart disease. If you are diabetic or pre-diabetic, it is important to work with your doctor to make sure you are getting the tests you need to understand where you are and what you need to do to manage your heart health.

MORE HEART HEALTH TESTS

HOMOCYSTEINE LEVELS: Homocysteine is an amino acid produced by the metabolic breakdown of methionine, an essential component of dietary protein. Recent studies indicate that elevated levels of homocysteine may be an independent risk factor for cardiovascular disease.

C-REACTIVE PROTEIN Another factor that may point to heart disease is a higher level of **C -reactive protein** which is produced by the liver and fat cells. It's level dramatically increases, when there is inflammation anywhere in the body, The higher the CRP, the greater the chance of a plaque rupturing and causing a heart attack. One thing to remember, is that CRP can be elevated for a number of reasons, If you are at risk for heart disease, consult your physician about having your CRP levels tested along with other tests to determine if a high level is actually in the arteries of the heart.

FIBRINOGEN: This is a sticky, fibrous protein substance manufactured by your liver that promotes clotting and is part of the body's natural repair system. A certain level of fibrinogen is essential and at normal levels fibrinogen performs necessary and important functions in the human body.. But too high levels can make the blood thicker and make it more difficult for the heart to pump this thicker blood through the whole body. There is also greater chance of forming a clot that can obstruct an artery. Many studies have shown that elevated fibrinogen is a risk factor for heart attacks and strokes. The normal range for fibrinogen is 200 - 400 milligrams per deciliter (mg/dL).

BLOOD PRESSURE MONITORING: Blood pressure is the measure of the force exerted by the circulating blood on the walls of your arteries. It is expressed by two numbers, systolic pressure (the top number, which measures the pressure exerted on the arteries during a contraction of the heart when the heart pumps blood out of the chambers) and diastolic pressure (the bottom number, which measures the amount of pressure exerted when your heart relaxes and the chambers fill-up with blood) High blood pressure exists when there is an increase in the amount of force needed to pump the blood through the arteries due to a narrowing of the blood vessel. The ADA recommends that for people with diabetes the systolic measure should be < 130 mm/Hg and the diastolic measure should be < 80 mm/Hg.

INTIMA MEDIA THICKNESS SCANNING (IMT): This is a non-invasive scanning technique, found by the American Heart Association to be a valid and reliable test for assessing sub-clinical antherosclerosis. A trained sonographer places a probe on the main arteries of your neck, and the images are then analyzed to assess the vascular health of your arteries. This test is an independent predictor of TIA, (stoke-like symptoms) stroke, and heart disease.

Waist circumference:
Waist circumference is one of the most practical tools to assess abdominal fat for chronic disease risk. A high waist circumference or a greater level of abdominal fat is associated with an increased risk for type 2 diabetes, high cholesterol, high blood pressure and heart disease. What is it about abdominal fat that makes it strong marker of disease risk? The fat

surrounding the liver and other abdominal organs, is very metabolically active. It releases fatty acids, inflammatory agents, and hormones that ultimately lead to higher LDL cholesterol, triglycerides, blood glucose, and blood pressure

Studies suggest that health risks begin to increase when a woman's waist reaches 31.5 inches, and her risk jumps substantially once her waist expands to 35 inches or more. For a man, risk starts to climb at 37 inches, but it becomes a bigger worry once his waist reaches or exceeds 40 inches.

To properly measure your waist circumference:

❖ The tape measure should be placed directly on your skin, or on no more than one layer of light clothing. •

❖ The correct place to measure your waist is horizontally halfway between your lowest rib and the top of your hipbone. This is roughly in line with your belly button

❖ Breathe out normally and take the measure

❖ •Make sure the tape is snug, without squeezing the skin.

The most important next step to take is to discuss your finding with your physician so that together you can plan a course of action to further assess your health and take steps to reduce your risk for chronic illness.

TESTING FOR PRE-DIABETES/DIABETES

FASTING PLASMA GLUCOSE: After an 8 to 12 hour fast, your blood is drawn and blood sugar levels measured. Per new ADA guidelines, A reading of less than 100 mg/dl is normal; 100 to 125 indicates pre-diabetes and 126 or higher is a sign of full blown diabetes. If your blood glucose level is abnormal after the fasting plasma glucose (FPG) test, you could have what's called "impaired fasting glucose. ("IFG")

ORAL GLUCOSE TOLERANCE TEST: During this test, your blood sugar is measured after a fast and then again 2 hours after drinking a beverage containing a large amount of glucose. Two hours after the drink, if your glucose is higher than normal, you have what's called "impaired glucose tolerance. ("IGT")

🔑 Although both IFG and isolated IGT indicate insulin-resistant states, they differ in their manifestation of insulin resistance People with predominant IFG generally have what is known as hepatic insulin resistance and normal muscle insulin sensitivity. "Hepatic" means "liver", and with hepatic insulin resistance, too much glucose is released into the bloodstream from the liver after a long period of fasting (such as overnight).

Individuals with isolated IGT have normal to slightly reduced hepatic insulin sensitivity and moderate to severe muscle insulin resistance where insulin produced does not work properly and in conjunction enough insulin is not being produced. Many individuals may have both IFG and IGT and manifest both muscle and hepatic insulin resistance.

HBA1C SCREENING TEST: A blood test that measures the level of Hemoglobin AIC in your blood. This test is utilized to indicate your average blood glucose over a 2-3 month period. Hemoglobin is the oxygen carrying pigment protein in red blood cells. It can react with glucose in the blood to form a sugar/protein complex called A1C which is a form of "glycated hemoglobin." (Glycation is a chemical reaction that occurs between sugars and proteins.) Once Hemoglobin A1C is formed, it remains in your body until the blood cells carrying it are eliminated. The normal lifespan of red blood cells is about 90-120 days. Therefore, the amount of Hemoglobin A1C in the blood at the time of the test gives an indication of the mean blood glucose over the past 3 months. This test is not a substitute for daily glucose monitoring, which is an important aspect of glucose control. Pursuant to ADA recommendations a normal HbA1c level is less than 6% for non-diabetics and a GOAL for diabetics is less than 7%. Studies show that people with diabetes who keep their A1C levels below 7% are less likely to have diabetic complications.

TESTS TO AVOID DIABETES COMPLICATIONS

DILATED RETINAL EYE EXAM: Over time, diabetes can damage the tiny blood vessels of the retina, (a light-sensitive tissue in the back of the eye that receives and transmits focused images to the brain) and abnormal blood vessel growth may occur. This condition is called Diabetic Retinopathy, a complication of diabetes. Retinopathy can be detected through a dilated eye exam performed by an optometrist or an ophthalmologist.

FOOT EXAMS: Peripheral neuropathy (nerve damage in the legs and feet) and vascular disease (poor circulation) are major factors contributing to diabetic foot problems. Together, these problems make it easy to get ulcers and infections that, without care, could lead to amputations. The best defense against these complications is tight glucose control, taking good care of your feet, and seeing your physician *right away* if foot problems arise.

MICROALBUMIN MEASUREMENT: This is a test that measures small amounts of protein in your urine. This test is important because diabetes can damage the tiny blood filtering units in your kidneys where waste products from your blood are removed and eliminated in your urine. This allows protein molecules in your blood, such as albumin to leak into the urine. There are no early symptoms, but your doctor can determine the presence and extent of early kidney disease by measuring the amount of protein in your urine.

THYROID TESTING: The thyroid is the body's accelerator, controlling the tempo of all its internal processes. When the gland doesn't work hard enough, a condition develops called hypothyroidism. When it starts to work too hard, hyperthyroidism develops. Thyroid disease is a leading contributing cause of high cholesterol, and left untreated, it can increase your risk of heart attack, stroke, osteoporosis, cancer and depression. Thyroid disease can be difficult to diagnose by symptoms alone because many other illnesses cause the same symptoms.

A TSH test can be taken to determine if your thyroid is working properly. This test measures thyroid-stimulating hormone, made by the pituitary gland to keep the thyroid under control. Criteria vary, but a TSH higher than 5 mIU/ml usually indicates hypothyroidism, and a TSH below 0.1 indicates hyperthyroidism. If you have glucose imbalances or diabetes you are at higher risk for thyroid disease and should talk to your doctor about testing. If your TSH test is within normal ranges, but your symptoms persist, you should consider speaking to your physician about testing the levels of the T_4 and T_3 thyroid hormones in your blood.

Your Personal Physical Inventory

You can request a copy of your blood work from your doctor. At a minimum keep a record of the following:

Date:		
Physical Measurements:		
	Height: Weight Body Measurements Waist BMI (Body Mass Index)	Within limits for height & age?
Blood Glucose Levels (Fasting Plasma Glucose) (Oral Glucose Tolerance Test)		Normal Range? Pre-Diabetic Range? Diabetic Range?
HBA1C		7% or Less?
Lipid Profile		
	HDL	Within recommended range?
	LDL	Within recommended range?
	Total	Within recommended range?
	Triglycerides	
	Other: (LDL-P) (sdLDL Levels)	
Homocysteine		
C-Reactive Protein		
Fibrinogen Levels		
Blood Pressure:		
TSH		
Eye Exam	Normal?	Follow up treatment required?
Foot Exam	Normal?	Follow up treatment required?

Other Observations:

Learn About Your Medications

Management of Type 2 diabetes may include oral medications that address two of the physical components of the disease: the inability of the pancreas to produce sufficient amounts of insulin and the inability of the body to utilize insulin effectively (i.e. insulin resistance).

If you are interested in adopting a more holistic approach to managing your blood sugar levels, it is important to understand what medications you are taking and how they work to bring blood sugars under control.

The chart below describes the various types of oral diabetes medications and the way they work in the body.

The information in the chart is provided for educational and informational purposes only.

You should always discuss the topic of taking medications with your physician, and you should not stop taking any prescribed medications without discussing this with your physician.

Type	Action:	Name (Generic)
SULFONYLUREAS	Stimulates increased insulin production in the pancreas	❖ Amaryl® (glimepiride) ❖ Glucotrol® (glipizide) ❖ Glucotrol XL® (glipizide ER) ❖ Diabeta® (glyberide) ❖ Micronaise® (glyberide)
MEGLITINIDES	Stimulates increased insulin production in the pancreas	❖ Prandin® (repaglinide) ❖ Starlix® (Nateglinide)
BIGUANIDES	Decreases liver production of glucose Increases sensitivity to insulin	❖ Glucophage® (Metformin) ❖ Riomet® (Liquid-Metformin) Extended Release (Metformin-Long Acting) ❖ Glucophage XR® ❖ Fortamet® ❖ Glumetza®
ALPHA-GLUCOSIDASE INHIBITORS	Slows the digestion of carbohydrates in the GI tract	❖ Precose® (acarbose) ❖ Glyset® (miglitol)
THIAZOLI-DINEDIONES	Increases sensitivity of muscle cells to insulin	❖ Actos® (pioglitazone) ❖ Avanida (rosiglitazone)

DPP4 INHIBITORS	Increases insulin secretion, Reduces glucose release from liver after meals	❖ Januvia (Sitagliptin) ❖ Onglyza (Saxagliptin) ❖ Tradjenta (Saxagliptin)
GLP-1 ANALOGS	Increases insulin secretion Reduces glucose release from liver after meals Delays food emptying from stomach and promotes satiety.	❖ Byetta (Exenatide) ❖ Victoza (Liraglutide)
COMBINATION DRUGS	❖ Decreases liver glucose production and increases insulin production by the pancreas	❖ Glucovance® (metformin glyberide)
	❖ Decreases liver glucose production and increases insulin production by the pancreas; also increases cell sensitivity to insulin	❖ Avandamet® (metformin rosiglitazone)
	❖ Decreases liver glucose production and increases insulin production by the pancreas	❖ Metaglip® (metformin glipizide)
	❖ Decreases liver glucose production and increases insulin production by the pancreas; also increases cell sensitivity to insulin	❖ Actoplus Met® (metformin pioglitazone)

Understanding Nutrients and Exploring Nutritional Supplements as an Adjunct to Your Medical Care

The LIVE FREE Blood Sugar & Diabetes Coaching System™, will teach you how to develop a food plan, as the foundation for controlling your blood sugars and reaching your health goals.

The best source of nutrients comes from the food we eat, and it is helpful to have a basic understanding of nutrition in order to select foods that support health and blood sugar control. Having said that, learning how every vitamin and mineral works is a complex topic that goes beyond what can be covered in this book.

In the following sections we will take a "1000 foot view" of how vitamins, minerals and a special class of nutrients called phytochemicals work so that you can use this information in developing your food plan and overall health strategy.

Depending upon your situation and unique biochemistry, it may not possible to get all the nutrients you need from food.

This section will also help you to understand how nutritional supplements can play a role in supporting better health when it is not possible to get all the nutrients you need from your daily meals and snacks.

Nutrients Overview

Food contains three primary components:

- ❖ **Macronutrients**: Proteins, Carbohydrates, and Lipids/Fats
- ❖ **Micronutrients**: Vitamins and Minerals
- ❖ **Phytochemicals**: Class of nutrients from plant foods that have properties that enhance health and fight disease, including helping cells repair themselves and acting as antioxidants to neutralize damaging free radicals.

MACRONUTRIENTS:
- ❖ **Proteins** form the body's building blocks and functional structures. Protein is broken down into amino acids which are used throughout the body to build & repair tissues & cells. *Enzymes* are proteins that "catalyze chemical reactions that are constantly taking place in our bodies to support various metabolic processes that sustain life.
- ❖ **Carbohydrates** are the body's preferred energy source.
- ❖ **Lipids/Fats** are the body's key energy reserve and precursors for cell membranes and hormones.

MICRONUTRIENTS:
- ❖ **Vitamins & Minerals** are essential to work with enzymes in our body (as co-enzymes and co-factors) so that enzymes can perform vital bodily functions that keep us alive and healthy.
- ❖ **Classifications include***:
  - ▪ Fat Soluble Vitamins: A, D, E, K
  - ▪ Water Soluble Vitamins: B Complex, C
  - ▪ Major Minerals: Calcium, Phosphorus, Potassium, Sodium, Chloride, Magnesium, Sulpher
  - ▪ Minor Trace Minerals: Boron, Chromium, Copper, Iodine, Iron, Manganese, Molybdenum, Selenium, Silicon, Vanadium, Zinc

PHYTOCHEMICALS

❖ **Phytochemicals** are nutrients from plant foods that enhance health and fight disease, including helping cells repair themselves and acting as antioxidants to neutralize damaging free radicals.

- **Flavanoids** are found in cranberries, strawberries, apples, onions, tea, cocoa and red wine. Studies show a link between a high intake of flavanoids and reduced risk of heart attack and stroke.

- **Cartenoids** are responsible for the red, orange or yellow color of many fruits and vegetables. Their presence is masked by chlorophyll in dark green leafy vegetables.

- **Isoflavones**: Soybeans are the most common source in human food.

How Vitamins and Minerals Support Health

❖ The role of vitamins and minerals is to help enzymes perform their function of catalyzing the chemical reactions that sustain our health. If an enzyme is lacking an essential vitamin or mineral, it cannot perform properly.

❖ A key concept in nutritional medicine is gaining an understanding of how to supply the necessary nutrients that allow enzymes of a particular tissue to work at their optimal level.

The diagram below shows an example of the synergy between vitamins and enzymes.

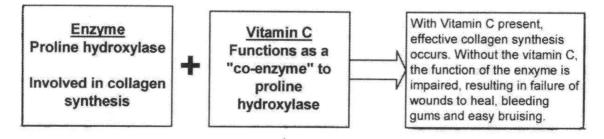

I eat a balanced diet, Do I Need Supplements?

❖ Fewer than 10% of the American population eats even the minimum daily recommended amount of plant foods: The minimum daily recommended amount of plant foods is five servings. It is not uncommon for individuals to think they are getting more vegetables and fruits than they are actually consuming. Check it out for yourself. Keep a food diary for a week to find out how close you come to meeting the daily requirements. The results may surprise you.

❖ Even if you eat well, the food you eat may not contain the nutrient levels that you need to maintain health, regulate your blood sugar levels and avoid serious complications of diabetes. Depleted soils, modern growing techniques, food preservatives as well as the cooking and refining processes all result in lower nutrient content of foods.

❖ More and more, experts are recommending vitamins: In a recent scientific review, two Harvard Researchers, Robert H. Fletcher, MD, M.Sc., and Kathleen M. Fairfield, MD. D.Ph. of the Harvard Medical School and the Harvard School of Public health, considered the evidence that less than optimal intakes of a number of vitamins are associated with an increased risk of chronic diseases. They stated in the June 19th issue of JAMA that "we recommend that all adults take one multivitamin daily."

Helpful Supplements for Fighting Diabetes

There is growing research and evidence to reveal that taking certain vitamins, minerals, and herbal extracts can have a beneficial effect on keeping blood glucose levels normal and avoiding the debilitating complications brought on by diabetes.

Although the kind of proof that mainstream medicine likes to see might not always be there, many experts are already incorporating some supplements into treatment regimens and others are beginning to acknowledge the possibilities.

You should not begin taking supplements without first discussing it with your treating physician.

Alternative healing techniques are a powerful, but complementary healing adjunct to conventional diabetes treatments. It is of utmost importance that you keep your health care team informed of any alternative treatments you plan to pursue.

If you are considering herbs or nutritional supplements, be sure to let your doctor know what you would like to try, and be sure to continue with medical supervision when you incorporate any new supplements into your treatment plan. Drops in blood sugar may result, and modifications in medication or insulin dosage may be required. Also, you need to know if a supplement will negatively interact with any of your other medications.

Do not be afraid to broach the subject of nutritional supplementation and to explore the possibilities with your health care team.

If your doctor is initially unwilling to discuss supplements with you, or is not familiar with a supplement that you would like to try, do some of your own research and provide the information to your doctor. Then, discuss your options as a team. Most doctors are willing to work with conventional supplements and to monitor your progress under their supervision.

If you would like to try complementing your treatment with supplements and for some reason your physician is staunchly opposed, you might try working with a physician that specializes in integrative medicine or whose practice involves providing a combination of conventional and alternative therapies for diabetes.

How Do You Know What Supplements are Right for You?

Everyone's biological makeup and nutritional needs are unique. Simple blood tests can reveal low levels of key vitamins/minerals such as vitamin D and magnesium. There are also newer genetic tests that can tell you what supplements may be helpful based on the presence of gene variations that influence a person's overall health. Additionally, there are now tests available that measure levels of selected vitamins, minerals, antioxidants and other essential micronutrients within your white blood cells called lymphocytes.

At the minimum you can assess your needs with your physician or other member of your health care team. On the following pages you will find a list of some targeted nutritional supplements that are worth looking into. The list is not exhaustive but is comprised of some of the key vitamins, minerals and herbal supplements that have been showing some promise in helping in the overall management of diabetes and its complications.

Vitamins & Antioxidants

Alpha Lipoic Acid	❖ Alpha lipoic acid is a sulfur containing compound that helps burn glucose, converting it to energy that powers your heart, brain, and other organs. ❖ Glucose is a potent generator of free radicals, which cause much of the cell damage and complications associated with diabetes. Alpha Lipoic acid is a powerful and versatile antioxidant that serves to protect the body against free-radical damage. It is almost unique in that it is both water and fat soluble, enabling it to enter virtually all areas of the cells to neutralize free radicals. ❖ Alpha Lipoic Acid has been demonstrated to improve insulin sensitivity and may help diabetics by facilitating better conversion of sugar into energy. By lowering glucose levels in the bloodstream and improving insulin sensitivity, alpha lipoic acid greatly reduces a major source of free radicals. ❖ Alpha Lipoic Acid shows promise in protecting individuals against diabetic complications, including improving diabetic neuropathy. Studies have shown that it reduces the glycosylation of proteins, improves blood flow to peripheral nerves and stimulates the regeneration of nerve fibers.
Co-Enzyme Q10	❖ CoQ10 improves energy production in our bodies and serves as an antioxidant. ❖ These effects are especially beneficial in the prevention of heart disease and cancer. Studies also show a benefit for improved glucose control.
Vitamin C	❖ Because insulin helps transport vitamin C into cells, diabetics are prone to having low intracellular concentrations of this vitamin, even if blood levels are normal. ❖ Vitamin C strengthens the blood vessels, especially the small capillaries, boosts the activity of the immune system, and helps protect against cardiovascular disease. Some studies suggest that vitamin C may reduce the accumulation of sorbitol in the cells, another probable cause of diabetic complications.
Vitamin E	❖ Vitamin E functions primarily as an antioxidant in protecting against damage to the cell membranes. It is comprised of compounds known as tocopherols, which are needed to protect the lipids, or fats, in cell walls from damage. ❖ Vitamin E provides benefit in protecting against heart disease and strokes. ❖ Some studies suggest that vitamin E improves insulin action and exerts a number of beneficial effects that may aid in preventing long-term complications of diabetes, especially cardiovascular disease.
B Complex Vitamins	❖ B3 is a player in many important functions, including energy production as well as the metabolism of carbohydrates and the action of insulin. ❖ Biotin helps the body metabolize carbohydrates, proteins and fats. It is thought to help lower blood glucose levels by improving insulin sensitivity while also stimulating the activity of an enzyme called glucokinase, known to play a role in the glucose uptake by the liver. ❖ B6, B12, and Folic Acid are shown to reduce the risk of cardiovascular disease. Vitamins B6 and B12 may also be beneficial in preventing diabetic neuropathy. ❖ Folic acid has been shown to help control homocysteine levels. Although all the reasons are not fully clear, there is increasing research that shows that there is a link between high levels of homocysteine in the blood and diminished arterial health.
Vitamin D	❖ Vitamin D regulates the absorption and use of calcium and phosphorous. New research shows it also plays a role in the regulation of normal blood sugars.

Minerals

Vanadium	❖ Vanadium has been identified as one of the few compounds other than insulin that can activate GLUT-4 transporters, in essence mimicking the action of insulin. (Insulin stimulates GLUT-4 transporters to rise to the surface of the cell and carry glucose inside.)
Chromium	❖ Chromium has been shown to improve the activity of insulin and to facilitate the uptake of glucose into the cells. Chromium also supports carbohydrate, protein and lipid metabolism.
Magnesium	❖ Magnesium has been shown to improve insulin production and response, thus further promoting optimal blood sugar levels ❖ In addition to the many functions magnesium performs in our bodies, it has a relaxing effect on the smooth muscle tissues that line the arteries. (resulting in improved blood flow, lower blood pressure, and a reduction in the likelihood of arterial spasms that may contribute to heart attack.) ❖ Magnesium can help decrease the risk of diabetic complications associated with arterial problems such as heart disease and retinopathy.
Calcium	❖ In addition to helping strengthen bones, calcium may serve as a protective factor against high blood pressure.

Essential Fatty Acids & Hearth Health

EFA's (generally)	❖ Essential fatty acids are a type of fatty acid that cannot be produced in the body and must be obtained through diet or supplementation. ❖ Following ingestion, EFA's are ultimately converted to substances called prostaglandins that act like hormones to help regulate a myriad of physiological functions, including cardiovascular health and fat metabolism. ❖ EFAs come in two common classes: Omega-3's and Omega 6's.
Omega 3	❖ Three essential fatty acids are found in omega-3 fats and oils: alpha-linoleic acid, eicosapentaenoic acid (EPA), and dosahexaenoic acid (DHA). ❖ Omega 3's provide a number of benefits including: relaxing constricted arteries, repairing tissue damage caused by clogged arteries, reducing levels of VLDSs (very low density lipoproteins, which are clusters of lipids linked to heart disease), lowering the rate at which the liver makes triglycerides, and stabilizing heart cells, making them more resistant to irregular beats that can cause heart attacks.
Omega 6	❖ The most important of the omega-6 fatty acids for the diabetic is gamma-linolenic acid (GLA). This fatty acid is derived from the EFA linolenic acid. ❖ You can get linoleic acid from vegetable, nut and seed oils, but many diabetics are deficient in GLA because they often have problems converting the linolenic acid to GLA. Without the enzyme delta-6-desaturase (D6D), omega-6's won't transform themselves into GLA. We lose D6D as we grow older and it is suppressed by a diet including a lot of sugar, alcohol, margarine or other partially hydrogenated oils. ❖ Supplemental GLA may be helpful in helping to improve peripheral neuropathy, which is caused by inflammation and deterioration of the peripheral nerves, usually in the legs and feet. ❖ Sources of GLA include evening primrose and borage oil.
Nattokinase	❖ An enzyme which has been shown to promote healthy circulation and reduce the risk of blood clots.

Herbal Supplements

Banaba Leaf	❖ Banaba leaf contains corosolic acid, a compound that has been shown to activate glucose transport into the cells, resulting in a lowering of blood glucose levels.
Garcinia Cambogia (HCA)	❖ Hydroxic citric acid, available as a standardized herbal extract of the fruit of the Garcinia Cambogia plant, inhibits lypogenesis, the process by which the body produces and stores fat and promotes more effective burning of calories. ❖ Garcinia Cambogia also increases serotonin levels. This can help to control your appetite, putting you in better control of what you choose to eat.
Gymnema Sylvestre	❖ The use of this herb for treating diabetes in India goes back more than 2000 years, and there is ongoing research into its effectiveness. ❖ Studies indicate that Gymnema Sylvestre may improve sugar control by slowing the absorption of sugars in the intestines. It may also help regenerate insulin-secreting beta cells in the pancreas.
Bitter Melon	❖ Bitter melon is a fruit indigenous to South America and Asia ❖ It has been shown to have a blood-sugar reducing effect, due in part to compounds contained in the plant, including momordica which is chemically similar to insulin.
Garlic	❖ In addition to enhancing the immune response, garlic has been shown to aid in lowering cholesterol and triglycerides and normalizing blood pressure, important concerns to anyone with diabetes or insulin resistance.
Flavonoids	❖ Flavonoids are potent antioxidants that protect cells from free radical damage and are beneficial for the tissues that take a beating from elevated levels of glucose and insulin ❖ Flavonoids strengthen the capillaries that are often damaged and fragile in diabetics. They can help improve blood flow to the tissues, particularly areas hardest hit by diabetes such as capillaries of the eyes, kidneys, extremities and the brain. ❖ One of the best studied flavonoids for diabetics is anthocyanoside, which is most concentrated in bilberry, a cousin of blueberries.
Fenugreek	❖ Preliminary studies indicate that the active component in fenugreek seeds, which are high in soluble fiber, may help keep blood glucose levels down by interfering with glucose absorption in the intestines.
Cinnamon	❖ New research is showing that cinnamon functions to increase glucose metabolism in the cells such that cinnamon may have a beneficial impact on blood sugar levels. ❖ Cinnamon also contains anthocyanins which improve capillary function.

****Any herbal supplement can possibly interfere with medications you are already taking, and you should ALWAYS consult your physician before incorporating herbal remedies into your diabetes care plan*******

📖 *Reflections*

For me, the addition of targeted nutritional supplements has made a world of difference in my ability to control my glucose levels with minimal medication. My daily supplement routine includes a general multi-vitamin, banaba leaf, chromium, vanadium, an antioxidant formulation, and Omega 3 fatty acids both from flax seed and high quality fish oil. I am grateful that my doctor was open to my trying this supplement program and was supportive in monitoring my progress as I introduced it into my daily care routine.

Suggested Reading and Resources

Navigating Change

The Power of Now: Eckhart Tolle, New World Library, 1999. Conquering diabetes requires living in the present moment. If you are stuck in the past, moving forward will be almost impossible. Worrying about the future and what could happen can immobilize you. The Power of Now provides excellent insights on how to make the most of today.

The Power of Belief: Ray Dodd, Hampton Roads Publishing Co., Inc., 2003.

The Miracle of Mindfulness: Thich Nhat Hanh, Beacon Press Books, 1976

Eating Mindfully: Susan Albers, psy.d., New Harbinger Publications, Inc. 2003

If emotional eating is an issue for you, these three books will help you to learn how to change long standing beliefs in order to successfully change behaviors. You will learn how to gain awareness so that you can transform your belief system and enjoy a more balanced relationship with food.

Health & Diabetes Coaching

Design Council-New Approach to Diabetes Management: Visit the Design Council's site to learn more about why health coaching is the missing link in managing diabetes. http://www.designcouncil.info/RED/health/#B4

Institute of Integrative Nutrition: IIN is the world's largest nutrition school, offering in-person education with the world's leaders in health and wellness. The school offers a cutting edge approach to nutrition that integrates and synthesizes the very best of eastern and western nutrition. You can learn more about their unique Professional Training Program at www.integrativenutrition.com.

Diabetes and Diabetes Management

Reversing Diabetes, by Julian Whitaker, M.D., Warner Books Inc, 1987, revised 2001.. Filled with excellent insights and information, anyone with diabetes will come away with a better understanding of this chronic disease and common sense ideas for bringing diabetes under control.

Dr. Bernstein's Diabetes Solution, by Richard K. Bernstein, M.D., Little Brown Publishing, 1997. Not everyone will be able to adopt all of the recommendations provided by Dr. Bernstein. But, if you are serious about conquering your diabetes, you will gain valuable insights into the nature of diabetes and how to manage blood sugars.

There is a Cure for Diabetes: Gabriel Cousens, M.D., North Atlantic Books, 2008. Based upon the Tree of Life 21 Day+ program, Dr. Cousens offers a protocol for successfully restoring the health of diabetics through lifestyle interventions, showing participants how a low-fat vegan diet can reverse diabetes.

Glycemic Index-Joseph Mendosa Web-site: Visit http://www.mendosa.com/ to learn more about the Glycemic Index and to obtain detailed ratings for various foods.

Food & Nutrition

Get the Sugar Out, by Ann Louis Gittleman, Three Rivers Press, 1996. There is no doubt about it, giving up sugar is not easy. A classic and forerunner to newer books about the pitfalls of sugar, there are so many good ideas in this book for eliminating sugar and substituting with other satisfying foods, you might find you don't miss sugar after all.

The End of Overeating: David A. Kessler, M.D., Rodale, Inc., 2009. Dr. Kessler's book unlocks the mysteries of why so many people are challenged by overeating. Dr. Kessler explains why we overeat when we consume foods that contain sugar, fat and salt, especially when these ingredients found in abundance in processed foods are manipulated in a certain way to stimulate our appetites..

Against the Grain: Danielle Walker, Victory Belt Publishing, Inc., 2013. Danielle Walker's cookbook is a treasure trove of delicious recipes that will guarantee you will not miss grains if you choose to cut back for better blood sugar control. Her book has over 150 recipes that are gluten free, dairy free, and grain free for everyday living.

Vegetarian Cooking for Everyone: Deborah Madison, Broadway Books, 1997. If you are not used to eating a lot of vegetables and whole grains, preparing them in a variety of ways can be intimidating. The winner of prestigious awards such as the James Beard Foundation Award for Excellence, the recipes in this book will make a vegetable lover out of anyone.

Get Cooking, Molly Katzen, The Harper Studio, 2009. The cover of this cookbook says it all, "150 simple recipes to get you started in the kitchen." If you are looking to learn how to prepare healthy foods in your own kitchen, this book will help you to make the switch from ordering out to making delicious, healthy foods at home.

Sensational Stevia Desserts, Lisa Jobs, Healthy Lifestyle Publishing, LLC, 2005. Although not officially classified as a sweetener, Stevia is an excellent and natural way to add sweetness to recipes that call for sugar. This cookbook is filled with a wide selection of delicious sugar-free desserts using Stevia as a natural alternative to sugar.

The Sweet Life: Diabetes without Boundaries: Sam Talbot, Rodale Press, 2011. Beautifully written and photographed, this is one of my favorite recipe books. Sam's message is that you don't have to give up eating well. If you enjoy good food, you will find lots of options in these nutrient rich recipes.

The Joy of Gluten-Free Sugar Free Baking: Peter Reinhart & Demine Wallace, Ten Speed Press, If you enjoy a "treat" every now and then and you are looking for grain-free and sugar free baking recipes, this book is for you. The delicious and easy to follow recipes will make a baker out of anyone.

Encyclopedia of Nutritional Supplements, by Michael T. Murray, N.D. Prima Health, a division of Prima Publishing, 1996. The world of nutritional supplements can be a confusing one. Michael Murray's book provides a wealth of information in an easy to read format so that you can begin to understand nutritional supplements and the ways in which they can support your overall conquer diabetes program.

❷ Implement a Food Plan to Control Blood Sugars

The days and weeks immediately after being diagnosed with diabetes or pre-diabetes comprise the period of adjustment we talked about in the change process section. Your mind and emotions may not yet have caught up with your physical reality. You will need to give yourself time to adjust and make changes in your lifestyle.

Many experts recommend giving yourself a year to fully adjust. But, you can't afford to get stuck in "analysis paralysis." Although you will need some time to put a full plan in action, you are obviously going to need to eat, and what you consume on a daily basis is going to affect your blood sugars.

So, one of the most important things you can get started with is developing a new Food Plan that both addresses the underlying causes of diabetes and controls your blood sugars.

Below is a summary of the Food Plan that will be explored in the remainder of this section.

LIVE FREE Food Plan™ Overview

Food Plan Success Strategies

❖ Eat a wide variety of foods centered around nutrient-dense non-starchy vegetables **(50%),** high quality protein, **(25%)** and small amounts of low glycemic index fruits, starchy vegetables, healthy fats, nuts/seeds, and non-grain based bread or other non-grain-based flour products **(25%) NOTE:** *you can reduce the amount of protein, just add in some extra non-starchy vegetables.*

❖ Choose carbohydrates wisely. Consume whole grains sparingly and avoid grain-based flour products.

❖ Eliminate all forms of sugar in your home pantry, and judiciously use substitutes such as Stevia.

❖ Increase fiber. (try to include at least 25-30 grams of fiber daily)

❖ Incorporate a moderate amount of high quality fats into your food plan

❖ Eat breakfast every day. (preferably within an hour of waking)

❖ Consume enough water. (and other healthy liquids).

❖ Adopt new habits that improve not just what you eat, but HOW you eat (Eat on as regular a schedule as possible, watch portion sizes, avoid overeating and learn to eat mindfully)

❖ Be prepared. (at home and out of the house).

❖ Create an environment that supports your food plan and vision of health.

Snapshot of the LIVE FREE Food Plan™

	Remember, there is no perfect diet. Honor your individuality, and learn to trust your instincts. Stay Hydrated with Water or Tea (Green, Rooibos, Black) WHEN IN DOUBT, CHOOSE WHOLE FOODS.			
EAT MORE:	# Non-Starchy Vegetables – 50% •Cooked or Raw •Green/Veggie Smoothies •Green/Veggie Juices Note: you can eat less protein, just add in some extra non-starchy vegetables			
	HEALTHY PROTEIN – 25% •Lean/Grass Fed Beef, Organic/Free Range Poultry, Lean Pork •Fish (Best: High Eco Rating, low mercury content, high Omega 3 content) Examples: Wild Salmon, Sardines, Herring, Sablefish, Albacore Tuna from U.S./Canada, Farm Raised Oysters) •Legumes (Soaked, maximum- one serving daily) •Tofu, Tempeh (avoid highly processed soy products) •Eggs, Yogurt, Kefir			
DON'T OVER EAT these nutrient rich foods:	**Small Portions - 25%** Starchy Vegetables Low GI Fruits Healthy Fats -Nuts/Seeds			
ENJOY Occasionally	Dark Chocolate (Sweetened with Stevia or 70-80% Cocoa) Baked Goods made with sprouted grains or Non-Grain Based Flour (Nut, Seed, Bean, Coconut) Stevia			
EAT SPARINGLY	Medium/High GI Fruits Cooked Whole Grains Sugar Alternatives (Sugar Alcohols, Splenda, etc.)	Fish with low eco-rating, high mercury, low omega 3 content (Example: Farm Raised Salmon) Highly Processed Soy Products	Dairy (cheese, milk, sour cream, cottage cheese, cream cheese) Saturated Fats (butter, any fat that turns solid)	Coffee
Totally Avoid	Grain-Based Flour Simple Sugars Aspartame High fructose corn syrup.	High fat, processed meats Fish high in contaminants	Trans Fats	Soda (Regular or Diet)

Putting the LIVE FREE Food Plan™ into Action

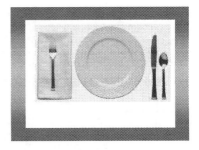

No matter how mild or severe your diabetic or pre-diabetic condition, developing and following a food plan that supports your physical well-being is the foundation for normalizing blood sugars and preventing or reversing diabetes complications.

But remember, your food plan is just one part of an integrated program, and all of your new lifestyle habits will come together to help you improve your health.

Why Diets are Not the Answer

The LIVE FREE Food Plan™ takes a "non-diet" approach to eating well for balanced sugars.

Developing your food plan is about building a self-motivated vision of how you want to eat to support your health. In a nutshell, you are determining *what* you want to eat, *when* you want to eat, and *how much* of certain foods you want to eat on a day-to day basis.

One of the big differences between the LIVE FREE Food Plan™ and a "diet" is that you are making your daily food choices based on a plan that is grounded in the context of both your physical condition and your self-motivated goals and long-term vision.

There are many reasons that dieting does not work for the majority of people, which explains why so many Americans experience yo-yo dieting and frustration. Below are some of the key reasons why going on a diet is not a helpful option to control or avoid diabetes:

❖ **Diets are temporary**: Most diets do not teach you how to eat for the life. Instead, they offer you a quick fix that is not attainable over the long term.

❖ **Diets distort your relationship with food**: Very importantly, diets teach you not to listen to your body. Instead, they instruct you to follow rigid menus, count calories, measure your food, and in general to ignore your hunger with will power.

❖ **Diets lead to boredom and frustration**: People often get bored or frustrated on diets and begin to cheat "just a little" and then soon abandon the diet.

❖ **When you diet you are likely to lose muscle and gain body fat**: When you go back to your old habits, you will gain back the muscle you've lost as body fat.

Dieting affects metabolism and puts you in fat storage mode:

❖ When you crash diet or cut calories drastically, you are temporarily slowing down your metabolism. This is because, when you eat less food than you need to maintain your weight, your brain thinks that you are starving and that you are going to die.

❖ Your brain misreads the lack of food as a life threatening time of famine. Your brain goes on red alert. It sends a message to your thyroid to slow down metabolism and conserve energy until food is plentiful again, thereby putting your body in a fat storage mode.

Dieting affects muscle loss and the ability to burn fat.

❖ When you subject yourself to artificial famine, your body considers itself to be under stress and the hormone cortisol is released in response.

❖ The function of cortisol is to quickly break down available sugars, dietary fats and dietary proteins in order to supply energy and spare fat stores for later use. If there is no supply of protein available, cortisol will take it from other tissues, causing muscle loss.

❖ Because fat is burned within our muscle cells for energy, studies show that losing even one ounce of muscle mass lowers the body's ability to create energy and reduces your fat burning ability.

❖ Ultimately, if old eating habits return, you gain back the muscle you've lost as body fat, which is why yo-yo dieters tend to gain more weight after each successive diet.

Dieting can result in a "double whammy" if you eat highly refined foods that put you in fat storage mode.

❖ We have learned that eating highly processed foods results in blood glucose spikes with a corresponding spike in insulin, and excess insulin throws your metabolic switch into fat storage mode.

❖ The combination of stress/starvation mode + high glycemic carbohydrates, results in more fat storage with a decreased ability to lose weight while high cortisol levels diminish your ability to burn fat.

THE BOTTOM LINE: Diets aren't the solution- they are part of the problem

Benefits of the LIVE FREE Food Plan™

The Plan takes a Non-Diet Approach: You are going to learn how to change your body composition through a healthy eating plan based on how your body works so that you can create a balanced physical state that allows your body mechanisms to function in harmony without following strict menus or counting, weighing and measuring.

The Plan is Realistic: Many programs are time consuming and hard to follow so that after a while most dieters give up. The LIVE FREE Food Plan™ is simple in its concept (eat more vegetables and protein, and go light on refined carbohydrates), and enables you to pick foods you like from a wide variety of sources.

The Plan provides long term success: You will learn how to eat in new ways so that:

❖ Your body's insulin response will be moderated,

❖ Your body will not store excess fat,

❖ You will maintain muscle that effectively burns fat,

❖ You will gain control of your blood sugar levels, and

❖ You will be supported in maintaining a healthy weight for the long term.

Tips for Making the LIVE FREE Flood Plan™ Work for You

As you work through this process, keep one thing in mind. A particular food is not inherently good or bad. **But, there are food choices that based on your particular physical condition lead you either towards or away from your goals and vision of health**. How you choose is up to you.

While many experts claim there are no good or bad foods for diabetics or pre-diabetics, the type, quality and amount of foods you eat on a daily basis **will** have an impact on your health and blood sugar levels.

The reality is that there is no perfect diet for diabetics or individuals seeking to manage a pre-diabetic condition. Everyone metabolizes food slightly differently. In the end you will know what works for you based on your own results (i.e. blood sugar levels based on daily monitoring, weight loss, your energy levels, etc.).

That being said, there are some guiding principles that will help you to manage both your blood sugar levels as well as cholesterol and triglyceride levels. Your food plan should also help you to maintain an adequate weight and provide adequate nutrients.

Remember, the guidelines set forth in the next section "Food Plan Success Strategies", are strategies for optimizing your food plan. They are not rules. The guidelines are meant to be flexible, and it is important to avoid a rigid attitude towards food that generally discourages the ability to stick with a food plan. With these guidelines in mind, you will be able to develop a daily food plan that supports your individual needs.

In order to develop the food plan that works best for you:

❖ **Keep it simple**: Any plan that is overly complicated will soon be discarded, and before you know it you will be back to your old eating habits. If you develop a simple, easy to implement food plan that is grounded in sound nutritional and behavioral concepts, you will find that before long you will start to internalize the plan, and making food choices within the context of the plan will become second nature.

❖ **Balance consistency with flexibility**: Planning what you will eat on a daily basis will enable you to avoid the pitfalls of impulse eating. The more predictable your food intake is, the more predictable your glucose levels are going to be, and the more accurately your medication and exercise needs can be tailored to support them.

❖ **Develop a plan that fits your lifestyle and supports your overall vision of health**: It is critical that your food plan is one that you are prepared to live with on a day-to-day basis, and so it needs to fit your lifestyle and particular needs. For example, if you are a vegetarian, you will want to incorporate ways of getting your protein from sources other than animal foods. If you have a hectic professional life or eat on the road often, you need to take these situations into consideration.

❖ **If you are diabetic, check your blood sugars about 2 hours after eating.** The bottom line is that it doesn't matter whether you are told you can or cannot eat a certain food. All that matters is how your body reacts to it. If your blood sugars are higher than they should be two hours after eating a certain food, it is not a good choice for you. Forget what the experts say, what is your body telling you?

Strategy #1: Eat a wide variety of foods centered around nutrient-dense non-starchy vegetables (50%), high quality protein, (25%) and small amounts of low glycemic index fruits, starchy vegetables, healthy fats, nuts/seeds, and and non-grain based bread or other non-grain-based flour products (25%) (to eat less protein, add in some extra veggies.)

❖ **Vegetables:** Filled with vitamins, minerals, fiber and antioxidants, fresh vegetables are critical for helping you maintain healthy blood sugar levels and steer clear of diabetic complications. Try to include raw and lightly steamed vegetables along with other preparation methods such as stir frying and roasting vegetables. Choose as many richly colored vegetables as possible. At least 50% of the food you eat daily should consist of non-starchy vegetables. Consume starchy vegetables such as sweet potatoes, yams and corn in moderation.

❖ **Fruit**: Fruits that are low on the glycemic index are optimal.

❖ **Greens**: Include at least one daily serving of deep colored leafy greens such as kale, arugula, collard greens, spinach or watercress. You can consume greens in a variety of ways, including in salads, cooked as a side dish, in green smoothies or in a delicious green drink/juice.

❖ **Grains**: For success with blood sugar control, avoid grains, or consume certain whole grains very judiciously. If you choose to include grains in your food plan, the best types of whole grains are cooked whole grains (quinoa, oats, barley, rye) or high fiber sprouted whole grain breads. If you are diabetic, you should check your blood sugars two hours after eating grains or grain based products to confirm their effect on your blood sugar levels. Avoid all grain-based flour products. (avoid gluten free flour made with potato or rice flour)

❖ **Protein** is an important part of your food plan. Your body requires 22 different amino acids in order to function properly. Eight of these amino acids are "essential amino acids" that can only be obtained from protein foods. The body can produce the other 14 amino acids from the essential amino acids that you ingest. You can obtain protein from both animal and plant sources, depending upon your lifestyle and preferences. If you include animal protein in your food plan, closely monitor the saturated fat content.

❖ When you eat meat, your health will benefit from eating **organic, grass fed** rather than grain fed animals. Meat from grass fed animals contains more conjugated linoleic acid (a component of fat that boosts fat burning and the buildup of lean muscle mass) and more healthy Omega-3 fats. Try to choose organic sources of both meat and poultry whenever possible.

❖ **Eggs**: Consumed in moderation eggs are a great source of protein and vitamins, including vitamin A, potassium and many B vitamins like folic acid, choline and biotin. Try to purchase eggs from chickens raised in a free-range or cage-free environment.

❖ **Yogurt & Kefir**: In addition to being a good source of protein and calcium, yogurts that say "live and active cultures" on the label contain probiotics that help maintain and restore the delicate balance of both "good" and "bad" bacteria necessary for a healthy digestive system. Kefir, a fermented milk product is also a rich source of probiotics,vitamins, minerals and essential amino acids/protein. Greek yogurt is lower in lactose and has twice the protein content of regular yogurts.

❖ **Legumes** are a great source of protein and soluble fiber, but be aware that they are a source of phytic acid, an anti-nutrient that binds with minerals in your gut making the minerals unavailable for absorption.. The best way to reduce the amount of phytic acid is to soak your beans overnight before cooking them. Try to limit the use of canned beans. Generally, beans should not pose any problems in the context of a well-balanced, nutrient-dense diet.

Strategy #2: Choose carbohydrates wisely. Consume whole grains sparingly and avoid grain-based flour products.

Of all the foods in your plan, the amount and type of carbohydrates that you eat will have the most dramatic impact on your blood sugars.

This guideline is the hardest one for most people to grasp and to follow. Understanding how carbohydrates work in your body will help you to make choices that will support normal blood sugar levels.

❖ Keep in mind that you are not going to avoid all carbohydrates. To the contrary, if you keep the following guiding principle in mind when selecting carbohydrates, you will rarely go wrong: "the longer your body has to wrestle with a carbohydrate to break it down into glucose, the slower the rise in glucose in your blood."

❖ The key to including carbohydrates in your diet is remembering that all carbohydrates are not created equal.

❖ You want to strive to include good quality complex carbohydrates in your food plan that are 1) unrefined, 2) nutritious, 3) high in fiber and 4) do not contribute to dramatic swings in your blood sugar and subsequent spiked insulin responses.

Carbohydrates 101

Hundreds of books, magazine articles, web-sites and diet plans have weighed in on the topic of carbohydrates. All of this information, much of it conflicting, makes it difficult for anyone dealing with insulin resistance, pre-diabetes or diabetes to make decisions about what to eat to bring blood sugars under control.

Diabetes is a core melt down in your body's ability to properly utilize glucose. As we have learned, your body must have glucose in order to survive, and carbohydrates are the primary food source for glucose. Unfortunately, a key characteristic of diabetes is the decreased ability or complete inability of the body to effectively utilize carbohydrates.

So, we start with the premise that everyone has to eat carbohydrates. But, if you are diabetic or have a pre-diabetic condition, carbohydrates have by far the greatest impact on blood sugar, so controlling the <u>quality</u>, <u>type</u>, and <u>quantity of</u> carbohydrates you are eating will ultimately produce the best blood sugar results.

In order to make informed decisions about what to eat, based on an understanding of your condition and how to use carbohydrates to your advantage, (rather than relying on the latest hype or low carb craze) you need to have a basic understanding of what carbohydrates are and how they are processed in your system.

❖ Your body gets the glucose it requires from the food you eat, primarily from carbohydrates.

❖ Carbohydrates are not foods but rather collections of molecules consisting of carbon, oxygen and hydrogen.

❖ Chemically, at their most basic level, ALL carbohydrates are made up of units of sugar. These sugar units are called saccharide units.

❖ Physically, carbohydrates take the form of sugars, starches, and cellulose.

- There are two main classifications of carbohydrates: Simple sugars and complex carbohydrates. Starches and cellulose are two types of complex carbohydrates.

- How fast carbohydrates that you eat on a daily basis enter your blood stream as glucose and the resultant insulin response has an impact on your health over the long run.

On the following pages we will explore how carbohydrates affect our blood sugars and how to select carbohydrates for optimal health. As you will learn, not all carbohydrates are created equal, and understanding how different carbohydrates affect your system will help you to make effective food choices.

Tips for Selecting Carbohydrates

Choosing to eat (or reject) a food based on the amount of carbohydrate it contains only gives you a small piece of the carbohydrate puzzle. In order to successfully manage blood sugars, a number of factors that should be considered, including:

TYPE ➜ PROCESSING ➜ EFFECT ➜ AMOUNT

FIRST: What type of carbohydrate is it? Carbohydrates fall into two main categories: **simple** and **complex** carbohydrates. Some complex carbohydrates like potatoes act more like simple carbohydrates in our system, and the amount of processing foods undergo also has a major impact on how carbohydrates affect our blood sugars. Nevertheless, understanding the difference between simple carbohydrates and complex carbohydrates is a good starting point when selecting which carbohydrates to include in your food plan.

Simple Sugars & Complex Carbohydrates

- Carbohydrates that contain only one or two sugar units are referred to as simple sugars. Simple sugars are often named according to the foodstuff with which they are associated, i.e. lactose (milk), maltose (malt, grain) fructose (fruit), sucrose (refined sugar).

- Simple sugars are sweet in taste and are broken down quickly in the body to release energy. This means they enter the bloodstream more rapidly causing a fast rise in blood glucose accompanied by a sharp rise in insulin to contain them.

  o Fructose is a simple sugar twice as sweet as sucrose (table sugar). Because it is mainly metabolized in the liver, fructose has a lower glycemic index. But, Fructose is incorporated into triglycerides more readily than glucose (blood sugar); therefore, it has a greater propensity to increase serum triglycerides.

- Complex carbohydrates are long chains of simple sugar units bonded together. As a general rule, complex carbohydrates are digested more slowly and moderate the glucose and insulin response. Starch and cellulose are two types of complex carbohydrates.

Starches are carbohydrates in which 300 to 1000 glucose units join together.

- Starch is a type of complex carbohydrate (called a polysaccharide) used by plants to store energy for later use.

- Plants store starch in seeds or other specialized organs, where it remains until needed for energy.

- During the digestion process starch is broken into soluble glucose units.

Cellulose differs from the complex carbohydrate starch because its glucose units form a two-dimensional structure, giving the molecule added stability.

- Also known as plant or dietary fiber, cellulose cannot be digested by human beings. (It passes through the digestive tract without being broken down by human digestive enzymes).

- Cellulose is a relatively stiff material, and in plants cellulose is used as a structural molecule to add support to the leaves, stem and other plant parts.

- Despite the fact that it cannot be used as an energy source in most animals, cellulose fiber is essential in the diet because it helps exercise the digestive track and keeps it clean and healthy.

- Additionally, fiber slows digestion, which has a beneficial effect on blood sugar levels.

Carbohydrate, Protein & Fats Overview

The diagram on the following page provides an overview of the various types of carbohydrates, fats and proteins and the types of foods included in each of those categories. The symbols included in the diagram are provided to give a visual rating of these foods based on their nutritional density and effect on blood sugars and/or heart health.

Symbol	DESCRIPTION
	Items with a bright yellow sun indicate foods that are considered by most experts to be healthful and nutritionally dense. Additionally, they are either helpful for blood sugar control or have little effect on blood sugar levels. Non-starchy vegetables get a really big yellow sun. You can't go wrong eating non-starchy vegetables, and for blood sugar control, they should comprise a major part of your food plan. Note that FISH has a yellow sun next to it because as a general rule fish is an excellent source of protein. (for those who are not vegetarian or vegan) But, it does depend on what fish you are eating. In general, you want to select fish that are have a high eco-rating, do not have a high mercury content, and have a high level of Omega 3.
	Items with a sun covered with a cloud indicate foods that have both healthy qualities and qualities that diminish health benefits. You don't have to totally avoid these foods, but they should be eaten in moderation. For example, legumes/beans are a good protein source and high in soluble fiber, but they also are high in phytic acid, which can affect mineral absorption. Many advocates of the Paleo diet say you should avoid all beans. But as long as you have a balanced food plan, eat beans in moderation and primarily eat beans that have been soaked before cooking, there is no need to avoid them totally and give up the benefits they provide.
	Items with a rain cloud indicate that these food items, although they are generally considered to be nutritious, can cause problems for blood sugar control and should be eaten with caution.(i.e. occasionally and in small amounts.) Corn and Medium/High GI fruits fall into this category.
	Items with a lightning cloud for the most part should be avoided due to their negative effect on blood sugar management and/or heart health. That doesn't mean you can NEVER eat a storm cloud food. For example, depending on your hearth health, small amounts of butter, Ghee, or coconut butter can be included occasionally in small amounts in food preparation. But be very careful with these food choices, especially if they are a trigger food for you and will sabotage your efforts. (For example, grain based flour products cause major issues for most people with blood sugar concerns and should be eating minimally, on rare occasions and in very small portions.)

Carbohydrates, Proteins and Fats Diagram

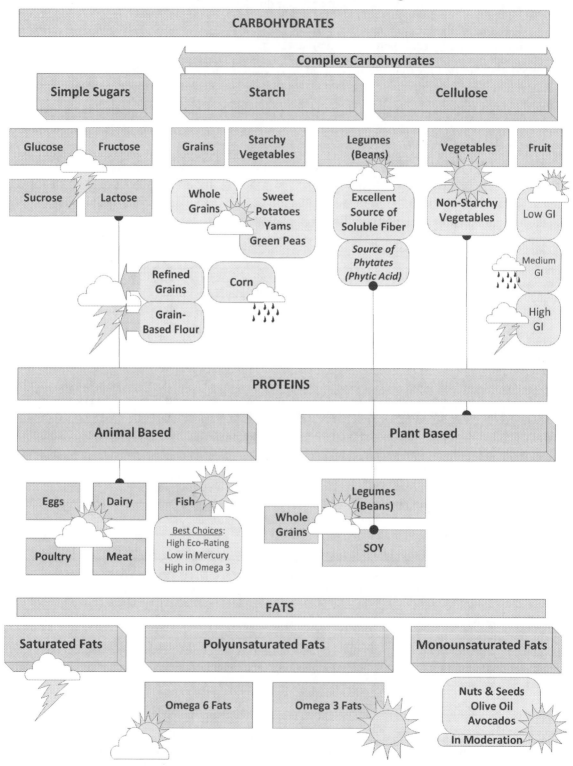

SECOND: What level of processing has the complex carbohydrate undergone? In general, you want to choose unrefined complex carbohydrates over more refined complex carbohydrates. (Examples: steel cut oatmeal or old fashioned rolled oats vs. more refined oatmeal flakes, brown rice vs. white rice, whole grain bread vs. white bread)

* Refined Carbohydrates are carbohydrates that have gone through a process that separates them from the minerals, vitamins, protein, and fiber that originally were present as co-worker nutrients that assist our bodies to metabolize them. Like simple sugars, refined carbohydrates are digested very quickly, and for that reason you should think of them as a hidden source of sugar in your diet.

* Examples of refined carbohydrates are white table sugar, white rice, and any type of grain-based flour. All of these products started out as unprocessed whole foods. Refined carbohydrates enter the bloodstream more rapidly, causing a fast rise in blood glucose accompanied by a sharp rise in insulin to contain them.

* Always try to choose an unrefined carbohydrate over a refined version. When complex carbohydrates are refined, the carbohydrates will break down in your system very quickly as if they were a simple sugar. In addition to the glucose impact, they are devoid of other vital nutrients. This is because the refining process separates them from the minerals, vitamins, protein, and fiber that originally were present as co-worker nutrients.

* *Avoid grain-based flour products*: Grinding grains into flour increases the surface area upon which enzymes work to more quickly convert starch into glucose. This means that any type of grain-based flour products have the same effect on blood sugar, whether the flour is produced from whole grains or not. Sprouted grain products are digested more like a vegetable with slower digestion and less of a spike in blood sugar.

* To metabolize highly refined foods, our bodies draw the missing nutrients from other sources, including other foods present in the same meal or the body's own tissues. For that reason, when we consume white sugar or white flour we lose B vitamins, calcium, phosphorus, iron and other nutrients, such as chromium from our own reserves.

THIRD: Consider the overall effect on blood sugar. Not all complex carbohydrates behave the way you expect them to. For example, starchy vegetables, like white potatoes, behave more like simple sugars, breaking down quickly into glucose and causing a sharp insulin response. Choose complex carbohydrates that release glucose more slowly into the bloodstream over carbohydrates that have a more immediate impact on blood sugar levels. This is where Glycemic Index can be helpful. For more detail on the Glycemic Index, see the section "Introduction to the Glycemic Index." Try to include complex carbohydrates that are higher in fiber and protein.

FOURTH: Consider the amount of carbohydrate when comparing similar food types. [Example: two brands of bread with the same amount of fiber]. As a general rule, when comparing similar foods, try to select the option with a lower net carbohydrate count.

Remember, not all carbohydrates are created equal. Do not lump all carbohydrates into one category in your mind, and be wary of any "diet" plan that does not take into account the difference in carbohydrates based fiber content and level of processing.

Strategy #3: Eliminate all forms of Sugar in your home pantry, and judiciously use substitutes such as Stevia.

For the greatest level of success with controlling blood sugar levels, the best course of action is to eliminate sugar in your home pantry, and consider it a marginal part of your food plan to be consumed very carefully.

I avoid saying never eat sugar, because, because for 99% of the population that is a recipe for failure, and your reaction to sugar depends on your individual biochemistry.

Finding Hidden Sugar in your Pantry

Sugar is the number one additive in the food industry. Each American consumes an average of 135 pounds of sugar each year. This accounts for 500 to 600 calories a day, amounting to over two pounds of sugar per week.

Refined sugar (white table sugar), simple sugars (including, corn syrup, honey, maple syrup) and refined carbohydrates (such as white bread and white rice) in general, place stress on our blood sugar control and other body control mechanisms.

Sugar and other sweeteners go by many names, so when you read food labels be aware of hidden sources of sugar.

Other names for sugar:

Barley Malt, Beet Sugar, Blackstrap Molasses, Brown Sugar, Cane Sugar, Carmel, Corn Sweetener, Corn Syrup, Date Sugar, Dextrin, Dextrose, Fructose, Grape Sugar, Grape Sweetener, Herbal Sweetener, High fructose Corn Syrup, Honey, Invert Sugar, Lactose, Maltose, Mannitol, Maple Syrup, Molasses, Polydextrose, Raw Sugar, Sorbitol, Sorghum, Sucanat, Sucrose, Sugar, Turbinado.

The Ongoing Sugar Debate

When high sugar foods and refined carbohydrates are eaten, blood glucose levels rise quickly, producing a heightened release of insulin. Keeping in mind that excess insulin promotes fat storage, it should come as no surprise that as Americans consume more and more sugar, government figures show that more than ½ of American adults are overweight or obese. This is an epidemic, increasing the risk for chronic illness and contributing to an estimated 300,000 deaths per year.

If you are diabetic or pre-diabetic, it is difficult to understand any logic that includes anything but very occasional inclusion of these refined substances in your diet when you have a disease characterized by your body's inability to metabolize them.

That being said, when it comes to sugar and refined carbohydrates, the experts are far from in agreement as to the amount of sugar to consume. Some advocate eliminating (as near as possible) all sugar and refined products from your diet, while others take a more middle of the road approach supporting moderation of sugar consumption and refined carbohydrates.

Unfortunately for diabetics, it is unlikely that the sugar debate (or the politics supporting the immensely profitable production of highly processed foods) will be resolved in the near future.

When you consider various points of view, keep in mind, as Porter Shiner notes in his book **New Hope for People with Diabetes,** "Yes, scientists have found that pure table sugar – sucrose – raises levels of glucose in the blood no faster than the starch in a piece of white bread, but this increase is still a lot, too much to allow sucrose to be consumed in large quantities."

There are other good reasons to stay away from the sugar bowl. In his book **Reversing Diabetes**, Dr. Julian Whitaker notes: "Some studies show a link between high sugar intake and chromium loss, which may also contribute to insulin resistance and diabetes." It is also important to remember that refined sugar provides no nutrients and can raise levels of triglycerides in the blood.

THE BOTTOM LINE: If you are currently consuming a large amount of refined sugar, or other refined carbohydrates, it will be beneficial for both your overall heath and your ability to control your blood glucose levels to eliminate or reduce your consumption.

The reality of our 21st century world is that most of us will include some degree of unrefined foods and sweeteners in our food plan. The key is to be aware of their effect on your system, to monitor your reaction to them closely and to try to keep them to a minimum. You will need to determine how and when you include refined sugar, sweeteners and refined carbohydrates into your food plan based on:

❖ your vision of your health and related goals

❖ your understanding of how these foods affect your system, and

❖ your physical condition.

When you are contemplating eating a food with sugar in it or other refined carbohydrate, be aware of why you are eating it (i.e. enjoyment, response to anxiety, convenience, boredom, etc). If you are repeating a pattern that led to your present condition and you are just substituting one sweetener for another (for example eating a whole box of "sugar free" cookies for a whole box of Pepperidge Farm chocolate chip cookies) think about how you can start to change that pattern to a healthier one.

The Problem with Fructose:

Fructose, also known as fruit sugar (levulose) is a simple sugar twice as sweet as sucrose (table sugar). But because it is mainly metabolized in the liver, fructose has a lower glycemic index. However, consumption of high amounts of fructose can lower metabolic rate and cause something called "de-novo lipogenesis" (the conversion of sugar into fat) since the liver can only metabolize limited amounts of fructose.

This means that a high consumption of fructose has a propensity to increase serum triglycerides. This is why I recommend closely watching fruit intake and avoid over consuming foods high in fructose, including Agave Syrup which has a high fructose content.

The Dangers of High Fructose Corn Syrup

There is one sweetener that many experts agree should be avoided at all costs, and that is the super sugar high-fructose corn syrup (HFCS). HFCS is an ingredient of almost every sweetened or processed food that many Americans consume every day.

When corn is processed into HFCS, this sweetener is absorbed more quickly than regular sugar and enters your cells, becoming an uncontrolled source of carbon (acetyl-CoA) that is the made into cholesterol and triglycerides.

Additionally, none of the normal controls on appetite are triggered when you eat foods or beverages containing HFCS so that you tend to stay hungry and keep eating more sugar and refined foods, which continues to fuel this cycle.

Diet Soda and Sugar Cravings:

A growing body of research indicates that drinking artificially sweetened diet sodas on a regular basis may set you up for weight gain and increased cravings for sweets. New research indicates that the body learns to predict caloric intake by the taste and texture of certain foods. When artificial sweeteners are introduced into the mix, our body sends the appropriate sweet signals to the brain but never delivers the sugar punch.

In this process we set ourselves up for cravings to which we eventually and often unknowingly, give in. In other words, consuming drinks that taste very sweet due to artificial sweeteners that seem real might be setting us up to eat more later on.

An occasional diet soda is probably fine. But, watch out for habitual drinking of artificially sweetened diet soda.

Kick the Soda Habit with this easy recipe for Lemon/Lime Spritzer

Sometimes you just want a sparkling drink with a hint of sweetness. Instead of reaching for a diet soda, which has artificial sweeteners and over the long term increases your craving for sweets, try this refreshing twist on the popular sodas 7-Up and Sprite. (For variety, you can experiment with other fruits such as Oranges or Strawberries, and you can try different flavors of Liquid Stevia as well)

Ingredients:

8 ounces sparkling water

2-3 slices of lemon and/or lime

2-3 drops Liquid Stevia (Sweet Leaf Brand- Plain or Lemon Drop)

Ice cubes (as desired)

Directions:

- ❖ Pour the sparkling water into a glass
- ❖ Slice the lemon/lime and squeeze some of the juice into the sparkling water, then add the lemon/lime into the sparkling water
- ❖ Add 2-3 drops of the Stevia to the sparkling water.
- ❖ Add ice cubes and enjoy!

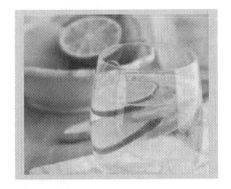

Quick Guide to Sweeteners

Common "Natural" Sweeteners:

Stevia is a non-caloric herbal extract with an intensely sweet flavor. It has been used for hundreds of years as a sweetener in South America and is a popular sweetener in Japan where it is put in everything from soft drinks to soy sauce. Until recently in the United States, Stevia was sold as a dietary supplement. Because refined Stevia is two to three hundred times sweeter than sugar, a few drops or sprinkles in your cereal or coffee are all you need. Stevia may also be used in cooking, but it does require some recipe modification in baking. Stevia is an excellent choice for diabetics as it has no calories, and it will not raise your blood glucose levels.

Agave Nectar is made through the extraction and purification of the juice of the agave cactus. Fructose is a simple sugar twice as sweet as sucrose (table sugar). Because it is mainly metabolized in the liver, fructose has a lower glycemic index. But, Fructose is incorporated into triglycerides more readily than glucose (blood sugar); therefore, it has a greater propensity to increase serum triglycerides. On occasion, it is an effective sweetener for diabetics, but should be used very sparingly because of its high fructose content.

Barley Malt, Brown Rice Syrup are sweeteners prepared by fermenting the grain from which they came. The fermenting bacteria convert the grain starches into simple sugars (and also some complex sugars) and still retain some complex carbohydrates. In addition, these grain based liquid sweeteners are a least half composed of nutrients that are found in the whole grains. Barley malt and brown rice syrup will have an effect on blood glucose levels and should be consumed sparingly by diabetics.

Fruit Juice and Fruit Juice Concentrates are fruit juices evaporated in a high vacuum using low temperatures until they reach a thicker consistency. Because they are so rich in flavor, it is often possible to reduce the amount of sweetener in your recipes. But, if you have diabetes, be careful and use fruit sweeteners very sparingly. They are still a form of sugar and will have an effect on blood glucose levels.

Maple Syrup is a natural sugar made from boiled down maple-tree sap. Pure maple syrup contains a full complement of minerals and is rich in potassium and calcium. If you are diabetic or pre-diabetic, you probably need to avoid maple syrup. Like refined sugar, it will raise blood glucose levels quickly.

Sugar Alcohols:

Mannitol, Maltitol, Sorbitol, Xylitol are actually neither a sugar nor an alcohol, but they do have carbohydrate calories, approximately ½ to ¾ the calories of regular sugar. Derived from plant products, the carbohydrates are altered through a chemical process. They are more slowly and incompletely absorbed from the small intestine than sugar, thus producing a much smaller and slower rise in blood glucose levels and consequently also a smaller and slower rise in insulin. But, it should be noted that the rise in blood sugar differs depending on your individual makeup, and some of the sugar alcohols may have a laxative effect. When considering products with sugar alcohols, moderation being the key. One exception to the common laxative effect of other sugar alcohols is the consumption of erythritol.

Erythritol is sugar alcohol that occurs naturally in a variety of fruits, such as grapes and pears, as well as in mushrooms, and. certain fermented foods such as soy sauce and wine. At the industrial level, such as for inclusion as an ingredient in Truvia, it is produced through a natural fermentation process. Fermentation is the process by which an organism metabolizes or "digests" one or more food sources to produce a desired product. Fermentation occurs naturally in a variety of different foods given the right conditions and is used to produce wine, beer and yogurt. In the case of erythritol, a natural yeast, Moniliella pollinis, digests a simple sugar (such as dextrose or glucose) and produces erythritol.

Erythritol is 60 to 70% as sweet as table sugar yet it is almost non-caloric and does not affect blood sugar levels. Erythritol has a very low caloric content; its value is 0.2 calories per gram for food labeling purposes in the United. This very low calorie value is due to erythritol's unique absorption and elimination process which does not require the metabolism of erythritol.

A major benefit of usingerythritol is that it is absorbed into the bloodstream in the small intestine and then for the most part excreted unchanged in the urine. Because erythritol is absorbed before it enters the large intestine, it does not normally cause the laxative effects that are often experienced after over-consumption of other sugar alcohols. Most people can consume erythritol with no side effects. Erythritol is commonly used as a medium in which to deliver high-intensity sweeteners, especially stevia derivatives, serving the dual function of providing both bulk and a flavor similar to that of table sugar.

"Combination" Natural Sweeteners:

Truvia: Truvia is marketed by Cargill Inc. The ingredients listed on the label are erythritol, stevia leaf extract and natural flavors. Labeling law dictates that ingredients be listed in descending order according to weight. According to the Nutrition Facts label, one serving of Truvia is 3.5 grams, and a serving contains 3 grams of erythritol. Erythritol is the largest ingredient in Truvia® natural sweetener by weight, and is used as an ingredient to provide bulk and the sugar-like crystalline appearance and texture for Truvia® natural sweetener. The erythritol used in Truvia® natural sweetener is produced through a natural fermentation process.

Artificial Sweeteners:

Sucralose: Sucralose, or SPLENDA® Brand Sweetener, is made from a patented multi-step process that begins with sugar (sucrose). Three hydrogen-oxygen groups on the sugar molecule are replaced with three chlorine atoms. Although the process for making sucralose begins with sugar, Sucralose is not recognized by the body as sugar or as a carbohydrate. It is not metabolized by the body for energy and does not affect blood glucose levels.

It should be noted that additional ingredients are added to SPLENDA® to give it volume and texture. These fillers include maltodextrin and/or dextrose which contribute a small amount of calories per serving. (less than 5 calories). Although widely used in the United States, there is some controversy remaining over the safety of Splenda which relates to the molecular makeup of sucralose. The sucralose molecule is an **organochloride** (or **chlorocarbon**). The root of the controversy is that while some industry experts claim the molecule is similar to table salt or sugar, other researchers claim that it has more in common with pesticides. That is because the bonds holding the carbon and chlorine atoms together are more characteristic of a chlorocarbon than a salt — and most pesticides are chlorocarbons.

Although some chlorocarbons are toxic, sucralose is not known to be toxic in small quantities and is extremely insoluble in fat; it cannot accumulate in fat like chlorinated hydrocarbons. In addition, sucralose does not break down or dechlorinate. So, the question remains, is Sucralose safe for everyday use? The answer is that we really don't know yet. The best advice is to use Splenda conservatively, in small amounts, if you would like to utilize it occasionally, and when possible use other types of natural sugar substitutes.

Aspartame, Equal (NutraSweet): Aspartame, the main ingredient in Equal and NutraSweet, is responsible for the most serious cases of poisoning, because the body actually digests it. Recent studies in Europe show that aspartame use can result in an accumulation of formaldehyde in the brain, which can damage your central nervous system and immune system and cause genetic trauma. The FDA admits this is true, but claims the amount is low enough in most that it shouldn't raise concern. The issue is for consumers becomes, to what degree are we willing to play Russian roulette with our health with by ingesting this type of potentially dangerous substance?

Aspartame has had the most complaints of any food additive available to the public. It's been linked with MS, lupus, fibromyalgia and other central nervous disorders. Possible side effects of aspartame include headaches, migraines, panic attacks, dizziness, irritability, nausea, intestinal discomfort, skin rash, and nervousness. Some researchers have linked aspartame with depression and manic episodes. It may also contribute to male infertility.

Saccharin: Saccharin was the first widely available chemical sweetener, Better-tasting NutraSweet took its place in almost every diet soda, but saccharin is still an ingredient in some prepared foods, gum, and over-the-counter medicines. The carcinogen warnings that appeared on the side of products that contained saccharin no longer appear because industry testing showed that saccharin only caused bladder cancer in rats.

Most researchers agree that in sufficient doses, saccharin is carcinogenic in humans, but the question remains pertaining to the level at which the danger occurs. That being said, some practitioners think saccharin in moderation is the best choice if you must have an artificially sweetened beverage or food product. It's been around a relatively long time and seems to cause fewer problems than aspartame.

Acesulfame K, Sunette (Sweet One): Acesulfame potassium is a calorie-free artificial sweetener, also known as Acesulfame K or Ace K (K being the symbol for potassium), and marketed under the trade names Sunette and Sweet One. Acesulfame potassium has been used in foods and beverages around the world for 15 years. The ingredient, which is 200 times sweeter than sugar, has been used in numerous foods in the United States since 1988

Tips for Cutting Back on Sugar

❖ First, cut back or eliminate the sugars you are least likely to miss. For example, instead of selecting a processed food that includes sugar in the ingredients, select a brand that has a small amount or no sugar.

❖ Stop adding sugar to foods, such as cereal and drinks, including tea and coffee (try Stevia, or another sugar alternative).

❖ Dilute concentrated sweeteners (such as honey with water), and mix sweet foods (for example granola) with an unsweetened food (such as plain cereal and nuts) to reduce the total amount of sugar consumed and to gradually get your taste buds use to a less sugary taste.

❖ Avoid "fat free" foods with high sugar content.

❖ Cut out soda, even diet soda, as some new research is showing that there seems to be a connection between the overconsumption of diet soda and sugar cravings.

❖ Try a combination snack of high quality protein and complex carbohydrate to beat a sugar craving. A few examples are nuts with a slice of apple, whole grain crackers with low-fat cheese, a turkey and lettuce tortilla roll-up with a touch of mustard.

❖ Get enough sleep and rest. When your body is tired, it wants energy, and that often translates into sugar binges.

❖ Eliminate refined sugar and sugary snacks from your kitchen. If they are not easily available, you will be less likely to eat them.

❖ Satisfy your natural desired for sweet taste with "sweet" vegetables such as sweet potatoes and onions. (Try caramelized onions on whole grain sourdough toast or mashed sweet potatoes sweetened with a touch of agave syrup).

❖ Explore the tastes of food without any added sugar, and use spices and natural flavoring extracts to add zip to your food. Coriander, nutmeg, ginger, cardamom, natural vanilla and cinnamon are all spices that can make a dish taste sweeter and help satisfy your sweet tooth without adding any sugar. Almond, mint, maple, coconut, and lemon extracts can be used to add flavor to everything from oatmeal to yogurt and sweet potato dishes.

❖ Do not restrict yourself to the point of causing a sugar binge. Incorporate fresh fruit into your food plan, and when you want to have a treat, go for one that has some health benefits, such as a good quality oatmeal cookie or a small piece of dark chocolate that is high in antioxidants.

❖ It is OK to indulge every now and then. If you opt to have dessert while out at a restaurant, split it with your co-diners.

❖ For a relaxing, energizing tea that also quiets sugar cravings, try the following sweet vegetable tea. [Bring 3 cups water to a boil, then lower heat and add ¼ cup onions, ¼ cup carrots, ¼ cup cabbage, and ¼ cup either parsnips or butternut squash. The vegetables should be cut in small pieces. Simmer covered for 15-20 minutes. Strain the tea and enjoy.]

Strategy #4: Increase fiber

Fiber provides tremendous benefits, both for the prevention of diabetes and for managing blood sugars for those who already have diabetes. Remember to start adding fiber to your diet slowly to avoid gas/bloating and build up to 20 to 30 grams daily.

❖ Fiber is the part of food that cannot be digested or broken down into a form of energy for our body. It is considered a type of complex carbohydrate, but it cannot be absorbed to produce energy. Fiber comes only from plants, fruits, vegetables, nuts, seeds and grains. No animal products contain fiber.

❖ Fiber comes in two forms: insoluble and insoluble fiber. While we need both types each day, soluble fiber appears to play an especially important role in glucose control. This is because it forms a thick gel that interferes with the absorption of glucose in the intestine, thereby reducing the ups and downs of blood sugar levels. It also helps to bind cholesterol in the intestinal tract, which is why it may help to lower cholesterol levels.

	Soluble Fiber:	Insoluble Fiber:
DEFINED	Technically called pectin, gum and mucilage, soluble fiber dissolves and breaks down in water forming a thick gel.	Technically called cellulose, hemicellulose, and lignin, insoluble fiber does not dissolve in water or break down in your digestive system.
FUNCTIONS	❖ Prolongs stomach emptying time so that sugar is released and absorbed more slowly ❖ Binds with fatty acids which are the building blocks of fat.	❖ Moves bulk through the intestines ❖ Controls and balances the PH (i.e. degree of acidity or alkalinity) in the intestines.
BENEFITS	❖ Helps to regulate blood sugar levels, lower cholesterol and remove toxins from your body. ❖ Slows the absorption of food after meals, thereby slowing down the conversion of carbohydrates to sugar. This in turn, allows glucose to be burned more efficiently instead of being stored as fat.	❖ Promotes regular bowel movements and prevents constipation ❖ Removes toxic waste from the colon ❖ Helps prevent colon cancer by keeping an optimal pH in intestines to prevent microbes from producing cancerous substances.
SOURCES	❖ Soluble fiber is abundant in beans, oats, barley, fruits and many vegetables	❖ Insoluble fiber is the roughage found in vegetables and the skins and outer coatings of grains, fruits and legumes

❖ In addition to helping to regulate blood sugars, fiber rich foods tend to be lower in calories and also curb appetite. A hormone produced by your small intestine stimulates a feeling of fullness that tells you to stop eating. The combination of nutrients and fiber in your food helps increase the production of this hormone and fiber plays a role in prolonging its presence in your system, thereby enhancing your satisfaction from food.

❖ The easiest way to ensure getting enough fiber in your diet is to follow the first food plan success strategy: Eat a wide variety of foods centered around a diet rich in high fiber nutrient-dense vegetables, low glycemic index fruits, and healthy protein. In addition to vegetables, some good sources of fiber include:

- o Flax: Always grind flax seeds before eating. You can grind your own or purchase ground flax seeds. Ground flax can be added to recipes, sprinkled on yogurt and salads, or included in your favorite smoothly

- o Nuts: If you don't have any nut allergies, include a few handfuls of almonds, walnuts, pecans, or hazelnuts to your diet every day

- o Legumes; Beans have high soluble fiber content and can be consumed in numerous ways. Enjoy them in salads, as side dishes or in your favorite chili recipe are just a few ways to incorporate beans into your food plan.

❖ If you are having trouble fitting enough fiber into your diet, try adding a fiber supplement. My favorite is Glucomannan which is a soluble, highly viscous dietary fiber a that comes from the root of the elephant yam, also known as konjac. Glucomannan can help you lose weight, lower your cholesterol, reduce your appetite, and lower your blood sugar. A good brand is PGX, which comes in a number of forms, including PGX Satisfast, a Whey Protein Drink Mix.

Strategy #5: Incorporate a moderate amount of high quality fats into your daily food plan:

In moderation, it is important to include certain "good for you" fats into your food plan. Among other things, fats are required for hormone production, facilitation of oxygen transport and calcium absorption, as well as for the absorption of the fat-soluble vitamins A, D, E, and K.

❖ Fats are made up of building blocks called fatty acids. The structure of the fat molecule determines whether a fat is considered saturated or unsaturated. There are two types of unsaturated fats in the foods that we eat: Polyunsaturated fats and Monounsaturated Fats. These are shown in the chart below:

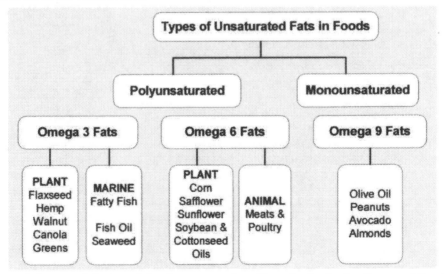

❖ Omega 3 Fats: and Omega 6 fats have opposite effects in the body. Omega 6 fats impede the benefits of Omega 3 fats, and if these two fats are not properly balanced in your diet, the overload of Omega 6 fats can dramatically affect your health.

❖ Omega 3 fats fight inflammation and keep blood vessels healthy by decreasing blood pressure and triglycerides, keeping arteries flexible and wide for smooth blood flow, and decreasing clotting and clumping of blood cells. Additionally, Omega 3 fats keep brain cell membranes healthy and fluid. Omega 3 fats from plant sources differ from Omega 3 fatty acids found in seafood. Plant sources contain ALA, which is known as a "short chain" fatty acid" that can be turned into EPA and DHA. These are the two longer chain fatty acids that provide the many powerhouse benefits of Omega 3 fats.

❖ High amounts of Omega 6 fats increase inflammation, blood clotting and insulin resistance. For optimal health try to limit the consumption of Omega 6 fats and increase your intake of Omega 3 fats. Most dietary Omega 6 fats come from salad dressings, cooking oils and spreads. One way to decrease your consumption of Omega 6 fats is to eat more monounsaturated fats which have no negative effect on Omega 3 fats and also lower cholesterol. Olive oil is the lowest in omega 6 fats. In moderation, nuts and avocados are also excellent sources of healthy fats.

❖ Limit the amount of saturated fats in your diet. Saturated fat raises levels of LDL cholesterol and increases heart disease. Depending on your condition, you can include a small amounts of certain saturated fat in your food plan, (such as organic butter from grass fed cows, coconut butter, Ghee, certain cheeses). But, always discuss this with your physician if you have a serious diabetic complication such as heart disease.

❖ The only fats that should be totally avoided are trans fatty acids. These are chemically altered vegetable oils that typically show up in foods as hydrogenated or partially hydrogenated oil. Trans fatty acids are commonly found in margarine, peanut butter, commercial snack and baked goods, and fried foods. These fats increase the risk of heart disease to a greater degree than saturated fats because in addition to raising total cholesterol, they lower protective HDL cholesterol. Growing research indicates that trans fats are connected not only to cancer, heart disease and aging, but also to immune system suppression and diminished ability to utilize essential fatty acids. Read labels carefully, and always choose products that don't contain these damaging fats.

Strategy #6: Eat Breakfast Every Day:

Do you find yourself craving sweets around 3:00? Are you still hungry after dinner? Do you find yourself snacking and eating well into the evening?

Believe it or not, what you eat or don't eat for breakfast will have an effect on how you feel and what you eat the rest of the day and into the night.

Also, eliminating breakfast can make losing weight more difficult. Why? Your brain uses glucose to function. If you haven't eaten in 6 hours or more, your liver will start to produce glucose. When you skip breakfast and become overly hungry, many people tend to crave sugar and carbohydrates and will now have an overabundance of glucose in their system, which ultimately turns into triglycerides, the pre-cursors to fat cells.

Some Interesting Breakfast Facts

❖ Eating breakfast within an hour can raise metabolism by 5-10%.

❖ Overall, eating breakfast helps to replenish blood sugar levels, burn calories more effectively and maintain more consistent energy all day long.

❖ At the American Heart Association's 43'd Annual Conference on Cardiovascular disease, it was reported that people who eat breakfast are significantly less likely to be obese and diabetic than those who regularly don't. In their study, researchers found that obesity and insulin resistance were 35 to 50% lower among those who ate breakfast every day compared to those who frequently skipped it.

Build a Better Breakfast

Everyone's biochemistry is different, and so there is no definitive e answer to the question, What should I eat for breakfast?. Having said the best breakfast foods are those that do not cause huge blood sugar spikes, set the stage for balanced blood sugars the rest of the day, and leave you feeling satisfied. As a rule of thumb, the more nutritionally dense the foods are t, the better you will feel.

Good Choices include: Healthy protein (such as smoothie with protein powder, salmon, eggs, turkey, low sodium turkey or Canadian bacon, hummus, tofu) with non-starchy vegetables

Optional: A small amount of healthy fat such as olive oil or avocado, or lower fat dairy

Occasional choices: high fiber whole grains, (sprouted whole grain bread or non-grain based pancakes/waffles/muffins/bread, cooked whole grains such as oatmeal or quinoa) and/or low glycemic fruit.

Breakfast Ideas

❖ *Breakfast Smoothie*: For a nutritious, easy breakfast, mix the following ingredients in a blender with a small amount of ice: Unsweetened almond milk, 1 scoop Vanilla Whey Powder, frozen blueberries. For added fiber add teaspoon of ground flax seed. For extra nutrition add a teaspoon of your favorite greens powder. Add small amount of sweetener of choice as desired.

❖ Cooked quinoa with almond milk, cinnamon, nuts and low glycemic fruit (such as blueberries)

❖ Eggs or tofu scrambled with vegetables of choice. (TIP: keep some sautéed onions in the fridge. Heat them in the a.m., and toss them into scrambled eggs. For added flavor add chopped peppers. broccoli, or sun-dried tomatoes)

❖ Hard boiled deviled eggs (if desired, substitute hummus for mashed egg yolk)

❖ Crust free mini quiche (with vegetables and cheese of choice)

❖ Yogurt with protein powder, berries and chopped nuts

❖ Almond butter/ricotta spread ½ sprouted whole grain English Muffin or piece of Paleo bread. To make the spread, combine 1 TBSP Almond Butter with ¼ cup part skim ricotta cheese and sweeten with sugar alternative of your choice. (add some protein powder or ground flax seed for extra nutrients)

❖ Turkey breast rollup with low fat cheese, avocado and sprouts

❖ Non-Grain-Based French Toast or pancakes with Easy Blueberry Syrup (For syrup: Combine 1 tbsp. No Sugar Added blueberry preserves, 1 cup of blueberries& small amount of water in saucepan. Cook slowly until blueberries are very soft & gently mash to release their juices)

❖ Smoked salmon, low fat veggie cream cheese, onion and tomato on non-grain based bread or sprouted whole grain bread

❖ Poached salmon with cucumber salad

❖ Hummus, avocado, red onion and tomato on non-grain based bread or sprouted whole grain English Muffin

❖ Stir fry with roast chicken and vegetables

❖ Tempeh or Turkey Bacon with lettuce and tomato

❖ Miso soup or other vegetable soup (with some form of protein included)

❖ Egg cooked over easy with slice of Canadian Bacon or low fat cheese

Strategy #7: Consume enough water. (and other healthy liquids)

Do you ever feel hungry soon after eating or tired when you know you have had a good night's sleep? Guess what? You may be dehydrated. Often drinking a glass of water when you have these symptoms will relieve the tiredness or feeling of hunger. Other signs of dehydration include constipation or dark urine.

❖ Water is essential for the proper functioning of every cell in your body and provides a number of important functions from lubricating joints, transporting nutrients to your muscles and carrying away waste such as carbon dioxide and lactic acid.

❖ Try to drink 6-8 glasses or water every day. (Note: if your kidney function is compromised or you have congestive heart failure, check with your doctor before increasing your fluid intake.)

❖ Green tea is another good choice, providing protective antioxidants.

Strategy #8: Adopt new habits that improve not just what you eat, but HOW you eat

When it comes to keeping your blood sugar under control, it's not just what you eat that counts; how you eat also matters.

Eat on as regular a schedule as possible and avoid over-eating.

❖ Eating regularly timed meals throughout the day, watching portion sizes and eating more slowly are all eating habits that put less stress on your digestive system and promote more level blood sugars. Eating at regular intervals also helps to avoid carbohydrate cravings that lead to binging when you let yourself go too long between meals.

❖ Watch portion sizes. One serving is approximately equivalent to:

Fruit & Vegetables	Whole Grains
❖ ½ cup cooked or raw veggies	❖ 1 slice bread
❖ 1 cup salad	❖ ½ cup cooked grain or pasta
❖ 1 medium piece of fruit	❖ ½ -1 cup dry cereal
❖ ½ chopped fruit	❖ 3-4 crackers
❖ ¾ cup vegetable or fruit juice	**Dairy**
Protein Foods	❖ 1 cup milk
❖ ½ cup cooked beans	❖ 4 oz. Cheese (4 cubes)
❖ 1 whole egg, 3 egg whites, or 2 egg whites with one yolk	❖ ½ cup cottage cheese or part-skim ricotta
❖ 2-3 oz. Meat, Fish or Poultry (approx size of deck of cards)	❖ 1 cup yogurt
❖ 4 oz. Tofu, ½ cup soy milk, ½ cup soy protein	**Fats, Nuts & Seeds**
	❖ 1 TBSP oil
❖ ¾ cup vegetable or fruit juice	❖ 2 TBSP nuts, seeds or nut butters

Don't let yourself get too hungry, angry/anxious, lonely, or tired.

Any one of these conditions is a set up for uncontrolled eating of refined carbohydrates.

❖ It's best to avoid these situations by implementing success habits such as getting enough rest and eating at regular intervals, as well as learning how to deal with your emotions, such as anger. Having said that, life is imperfect, and there will be times when you are very hungry, very tired, extremely angry or feeling lonely.

❖ When you find yourself in one of these situations, have a plan for acting in a positive way rather than reacting to your feelings by eating foods that will cause your blood sugars to spike. For example, line up a friend that you know you can call at times when you are angry or upset. Or, for times when you are feeling frazzled and tempted to sooth yourself with food, keep a list on your refrigerator of 10 things you would rather do than eat. Always keep healthy snacks available for those times when you go too long between meals.

Eat Mindfully

❖ Eat Mindfully, meaning make a connection with your food by breaking mindless eating routines, such as eating in front of the TV or eating while multi-tasking or when you are bored.

❖ When you are eating mindlessly, you are barely aware of what you are eating, and this can lead to overeating and having problems with portion control. In this state, you are moving on to the next bite before you have experienced the bite that you have in your mouth.

Benefits of Mindful Eating

When you slow down enough to taste and enjoy food, you:

❖ begin to enjoy what you eat,

❖ eat less, and

❖ make better decisions about what to eat.

Mindfulness Exercise:

What is your general state of mind when you are eating? Which statements below most apply to you?

❑ Most often I am mindlessly unaware, multi-tasking when eating, and unaware of portion sizes, (for example eating directly out of a bag of or standing in front of the refrigerator eating)

❑ Most often I am eating rapidly, Taking big bites, I tend to finish everything on my plate.

❑ Most often I am very inattentive to what I am eating, not really tasting the food.

❑ Sometimes I am aware of portion sizes. Occasionally I notice taste, texture and smell of my food

❑ Sometimes I am alert. 25 % of my eating experience I chew my food several times and my attention is directed to eating

❑ I make a conscious effort to be mindfully aware when I eat. I chew at least 25 times when I eat or at the very least I am aware of every bite and full chew it before swallowing. I pay attention to the sensations of the food I am eating. I enjoy every bite.

Tips for Mindful Eating:

❖ **Heighten your awareness of what you are eating**: This means slowing down when you eat, paying attention to what you are eating, and really tasting and enjoying your food.

❖ **Become aware of mindless eating**: Here are some common reasons that people engage in mindless eating. Be aware if any of these apply when you are eating food. Don't beat yourself up if you find yourself eating for reasons other than hunger for food, becoming aware is a first step towards changing habitual eating habits.

  o To relieve boredom or stress

  o To find comfort in tough situations

  o To quiet negative thoughts or to numb emotions

  o Out of habit (example: to use food as a reward or to eat while watching TV)

  o To navigate social situations (such as mindlessly eating at a party when you aren't really hungry)

❖ **Become aware of your food triggers**. What emotions push you to eat? What thoughts or environmental factors trigger eating, especially snacks and sweets?

❖ **Stop or limit multitasking when you eat**. Giving your food your complete attention enables you to connect with your body and supports eating out of hunger not to feed your emotions.

Strategy #9: Be Prepared in and out of the house

Sticking to your food plan outside of your home environment involves one cardinal rule that you need to follow religiously: **Take Care of Yourself**.

You don't have to eat Aunt Mary's birthday cake to make her happy, you don't have to eat the white dinner rolls just because the waiter brought them to the table, and you CAN ask what is in the sauce on the salmon and request that it be brought on the side.

Start to think outside the box and let go of worrying what everyone else will think. Remember, it's your life, and no one will take care of it but you.

Eating Out

If you think ahead and plan for outside activities, you can take care of yourself without feeling deprived. The two most dangerous traps for people with blood sugar issues when eating out are the bread basket, starchy sides (potatoes and rice) and dessert.

❖ If you are eating with a group, as soon as you sit down, when the waiter is taking drink orders, ask for a soup or salad to be brought right away so you have something to eat while others are eating bread.

❖ If you want to enjoy some bread with the rest of the group, plan ahead and bring some gourmet sprouted bread or bread made with non-grain-based flour to dip in olive oil.

❖ If you are eating alone, tell the serer not to bring any bread to the table.

❖ Skip the potatoes and ask for a double helping of vegetables.

❖ Avoid foods dipped in batter and fried foods.

❖ Enjoy a piece of Stevia sweetened or 80% Cocoa dark chocolate to enjoy with a frothy cappuccino for dessert

Healthy Snacking

Keep a stash of healthy snacks at your desk or the office fridge. If your office doesn't have a shared refrigerator, invest in a small lunch bag that has an ice pack that can be refreshed or some other type of container that can keep food cold for the day.

Snack Suggestions

❖ Pumpkin Seed Mix (1/4 cup)

❖ ¼ cup nuts (almonds, walnuts, pecans) with a slice of low fat cheese or raw veggies.

❖ 1 TBSP almond butter with a piece of non-grain based bread or apple slices

❖ Low fat goat cheese with Cherry Tomatoes

❖ Turkey rollups with avocado

❖ Chopped tomato salad with avocado and Italian Dressing

❖ .Cherry tomatoes with tuna salad

❖ Deviled egg (if desired, with hummus substituted for mashed egg yolk)

❖ Hummus or Bean Dip with raw vegetables

❖ ¼ cup part skim ricotta cheese with unsweetened cocoa and a tablespoon of chocolate protein powder. (Add Stevia or Truvia to taste.)

❖ Cucumber or zucchini rounds with hummus or tuna salad

❖ Spicy, Roasted Chick Peas

❖ Guacamole with Jicama sticks

❖ Cup of lentil, vegetable or black bean soup.

❖ Sardines with balsamic marinated onions

❖ Baby spinach "rollups" with Laughing Cow Cheese and walnuts

Strategy #10: Create an environment that supports your vision of health.

❖ The old sayings "your home is your castle" and "the kitchen is the heart of the home" have special meaning when you are trying to deal with diabetes, pre-diabetes or losing weight. You can't control the rest of the world, but you can create a safe and supportive environment in your own home where your surroundings enhance your ability to stay on track and maintain control of your blood glucose levels.

❖ A well-stocked pantry takes the stress out of meal planning and prep because it ensures that you have everything you need to put together foods that support your health, even if you are too busy to get to the store everyday

❖ The Empowered Pantry Makeover™ set forth in the following pages will provide you with guidelines for creating a kitchen that is a place where you can go to feel restored and experience vibrant health. You will also learn about foods and ingredients that will sabotage your efforts, how to recognize them, and the foods you can use as healthy alternatives.

The Crave Control Kitchen™ Makeover

Step #1: READ LABELS to find out what is in your pantry.

❖ It is not necessary to complete your kitchen makeover all at once. In fact for most people that would be expensive and foreboding. So, the first step is taking stock of what you currently have in your kitchen.

❖ Be your own food advocate by becoming a "Food Detective". Don't fall for fancy food marketing. The food label will tell you everything you need to know about the contents of any processed food.

❖ Getting Started: Go through your kitchen with a pen and paper & make note of all products you want to Remove & Replace. In Steps 2 & # you will remove unwanted foods and replace them with blood sugar friendly alternatives. In Step 4, you will learn how to totally restock your pantry.

❖ Food labels have both a Nutrition Facts and an Ingredients section, which provide different types of information. Below is a sample label for a typical whole wheat bread. The content is prepared by the food manufacturer's nutritional department.

Store Brand Wheat Bread	
Serving Size 2 Slices (47 Grams)	
Servings Per Container about 12	
Amount Per Serving	
%Daily Values based on 2000 calorie daily diet	
Calories 130	Calories from Fat 20
Total Fat	0.2g (3%)
Saturated Fat	0 g (0%)
Trans Fat	0 g
Cholesterol	0mg (0%)
Sodium	230mg (55)
Total Carbohydrate	15g (5%)
Dietary Fiber	2g (8%)
Soluble Fiber	(not calculated)
…Insoluble Fiber	(not calculated)
Sugars	3g
Protein	4g
Vitamin a 0%	Vitamin C 0%
Calcium 6%	Iron 10%
Thiamin 15%	Riboflavin 8%
Niacin 10%	Folic Acid 15%
Calories Per Gram	
Fat 9 Carbohydrate 4 Protein 4	
INGREDIENTS: Enriched Wheat Flour (flour malted barley flour), Iron, Niacin, Thiamin Mononitrate (Vitamin B1), Riboflavin (Vitamin B2), Folic Acid, Water, Whole Wheat Flour, High Fructose Corn Syrup, Yeast, Wheat Bran, Soybean Oil, Salt, What Gluten, Mono- and Diglycerides, Calcium Propionate, Datem, Calcium Phosphate, Soy Lecithin, Soy Flour	

Below is an explanation of the basic food label contents:

- **Label Contents**: Always read both the Nutrition Facts and Ingredients sections of the Food Label to understand the health value of a food product. Together, they give you the TRUE picture as to the health & nutritional value of the food product

- **Ingredients**: are listed in order, starting with the ingredient found in the largest amount, by weight, and progressing to the ingredient present in the smallest amount.. If the list of ingredients is long with words you don't recognize, it is likely that there are artificial and chemical ingredients that you want to avoid.

- **Serving Size**: : Reflects the amount that the average person eats at one helping. This amount is set by the F.D.A., for all similar products. Calorie counts are always by serving size, so make sure that you read the serving size carefully.

- **Calories**: Reflects the calories per serving. In the label above, 1 slice of bread would be 75 calories. (1 serving = 2 slices of bread and 1 serving = 130 Calories)

- **Dietary Fiber**: tells you how many grams of fiber are in one serving. Some labels will also give you the breakdown if soluble and insoluble fiber.

- **Total Fat**: tells you how many grams of fat are in one serving. All Fats MUST be listed. Here we see that there are .2 g of Fat per serving, But looking at Saturated fat (0g) and Trans Fats (0g) it appears that the fat is NOT a saturated or Trans Fat. The only way to tell the source of the fat is to read the Ingredients, which lists Soybean Oil as the fat source. NOTE: In the U.S., if a food has less than 0.5 grams of trans fat per serving, the food label can read 0 grams trans fat, which means you need to check the Ingredients to see if there are any "partially hydrogenated oils or shortening in the food.

- **Trans Fats** will be specifically shown on the label if more than .05 grams are present. If a label says 0 grams Trans Fats, check the Ingredients for the words "partially hydrogenated" or "shortening, which indicate that the food item does contain Trans Fats.

- **Sodium**: Sets forth the total amount of sodium per serving. Generally look for canned goods with reduced sodium content.

- **Total Carbohydrate**: Reflects the total amount of carbohydrates in the food product. In the label above, the amount is 15g, not high for two slices. BUT, note that the first ingredient is enriched Wheat Flour (Always read the ingredients to determine if the food product contains flour, and if so the source. (avoid grain-based flour and gluten free products with highly processed potato or rice flour) Sprouted grain breads/products contain whole grains, but do not contain flour.

- **Sugar** Lists the amount of all sugar. The source can be natural sugar from the food itself or added sugar. . (examples: sugar, dextrose, maple syrup, honey, fructose) The way to tell is to read the ingredients. As a general rule, you want to avoid food products with ADDED sugar listed in the ingredients in an amount over 1 gram as well as foods with large amounts of naturally occurring sugar.

STEP #2: REMOVE items that do not support blood sugar control

The idea behind removing certain items from your pantry is two-fold.

First, if the items are not readily available in your home, it will make it easier not to eat these foods that don't support your health.

Second, the one thing you can control is your home eating environment. Eliminating these items from your pantry doesn't mean you will never eat them. They are foods that you may choose to eat sparingly when you are out or in restaurants on occasion.

For Vibrant Health and Blood Sugar Control, ELIMINATE:

❖ **Food products containing Trans Fatty Acids**. Trans Fats will be listed in the Nutritional Facts section if more than .05 grams are present. If a label says 0 grams Trans Fats, check the Ingredients for the words "partially hydrogenated" or "shortening", which indicate that the food item does contain Trans Fats.

❖ **Products containing high fructose corn syrup**

❖ **Products with high amounts of *added sugar***. Generally, where sugar is one of the first ingredients, the product should be avoided. If the sugar content is over 1-2 grams, read the Ingredients to determine if the product contains *added sugars* and eliminate products with added sugars over 1g

❖ **Grain-based flour products**, including bread, crackers, cereals or pasta made with grain-based flour.

❖ **White Rice**, (Even brown rice may be too high glycemic for some people)

❖ **White Potatoes** (white potatoes, behave more like simple sugars, breaking down quickly into glucose and causing a sharp insulin response)

❖ **High sodium processed foods,** including high sodium canned foods and meat products

Below are some additional tips for cleaning out your pantry

❖ You don't need to eliminate all foods with saturated fats. But, you should be mindful and carefully consider both the source and the amount.

❖ Be careful with fructose in any form. (Eliminate high glycemic fruits, such as raisins)

❖ Avoid products containing nitrates

❖ Eliminate trigger foods. These are foods trigger you to keep eating beyond a small portion or to eat another food that spikes blood sugars. Potato and tortilla chips are examples of foods that some people can't put down. There is no harm in eating a few chips every now and again. But if you will eat half the bag in one sitting, it is best if they are not in your kitchen pantry. Chocolate is another problem food for many. Some people can eat a small piece of dark chocolate and be satisfied. But if you are a person that must eat the whole chocolate bar at one sitting, chocolate is not for you. Another category of trigger foods are foods that lead to another food that spikes blood sugars. For example, if a cup of coffee is a trigger for you to have a few cookies, then avoid coffee and substitute a non-trigger hot drink. Paleo pancakes are OK on occasion, but if you find that pancakes trigger a strong desire for maple syrup, they are best avoided.

STEP #3: REPLACE discarded items with alternatives that support blood sugar control

Substitutions Guide

Instead of:	Try:
Refined Sugar	Stevia, Xylitol, Erythritol, Brown Rice Syrup (sparingly)
White or Bread containing grain-based flour	Paleo Bread (Store bought or Homemade); Sprouted Grain Bread,
White Rice	Cauliflower Rice, Barley, Quinoa, (watch portion sizes)
Risotto	Substitute barley or quinoa for Arborio rice
Crackers	Wasa Crispbreads, Ryvita, Mestemacher Bread (whole grain rye); Cucumber or zucchini rounds
Sugar laden jams & jellies	Fruit Juice sweetened. Good choices include jams and jellies from Sorrel Ridge, Bionaturae®, and Kozlowski Farms.
Polyunsaturated vegetable oils	Olive Oil (watch cooking temperature when cooking with Olive Oil)
Salad dressings with sugar in the ingredients	Homemade with olive oil or sugar free choices such as Newman's Own® Olive Oil and Vinegar Dressing, Annie's Naturals Organic Olive Oil Vinaigrette., Trader Joe's Olive Oil and Red Wine Vinegar
Marinades containing sugar	Drew's® All Natural Salad Dressings and 10 Minute Marinades
Ketchup	Mustard (experiment with different types and flavors-sugar free)
Baked Goods	Baked goods made with non-grain flour (avoid potato or rice)
Chocolate Candy	Lily's® or Coco Polo® Dark Chocolate, (Sweetened with Stevia & Erythritol)
Cream Cheese	Spreadable Goat Cheese (Soignon is an excellent brand)
Excessive salt	Substitute Braggs Amino Acids for soy sauce/tamari; experiment with salt free spice mixes (Trader Joes 21 Salute is excellent)
Potato Chips	Nuts, Seeds, Sprouted Grain pretzels, roasted seaweed (seasnax®)
Fries with a Sandwich	Coleslaw, pickles, marinated vegetables, small salad
Soda, Diet Soda	Sparkling Water with Lemon/Lime (or orange slices)Sweetened with Stevia. (flavored or powder)
Ice cream	Plain Yogurt or Part Skim Ricotta flavored with Cinnamon, Vanilla and Truvia or Stevia. (add flavored Whey Powder for extra protein)
Milkshakes	Smoothies (vanilla unsweetened almond milk, whey powder, , frozen blueberries, almond butter, flax seed), Mocha Freeze (½ cup coffee with ½ cup ice, 1-2 scoops chocolate protein powder, low fat milk or almond milk) Add Truvia or Stevia for additional sweetness
Cold Cereal	Quinoa Porridge, Steel Cut Oatmeal, Oat Bran

STEP #4: RE-STOCK your pantry with new items that support your ability to easily prepare delicious healthy, meals and snacks that support your health goals

The Crave Control Kitchen™ Shopping Guide

The list is not exhaustive nor is it necessary to have every item mentioned. The idea is to always have food and staples available so that you can avoid making last minute food choices that don't support your overall health.

Low GI, Non Starchy Vegetables

For optimum health, try to include 5-9 servings daily. To get the most health benefits from eating vegetables, eat both raw and cooked vegetables and include a rainbow of colors. Include leafy dark greens daily.

Vegetables provide a wide range of nutrients such as vitamins, minerals and carbohydrates. They are an excellent source of *antioxidants* (substances that protect the body by neutralizing free radicals, which can damage cells) as well as *phytochemicals* (the bioactive compounds in plants that give them their color and flavor and provide many health benefits associated with eating vegetables).

❖	Red:	Red Peppers, Radishes, Radicchio, Red Onions, Rhubarb, Tomatoes (whole and small cherry)
❖	Yellow/Orange	Yellow Peppers, Rutabagas, Yellow Summer Squash, Carrots, Spaghetti Squash
❖	White	Cauliflower, Garlic, Ginger, Jerusalem Artichokes, Jicama, Kohlrabi, Mushrooms, Onions, Shallots
❖	Green	Artichokes, Arugula, Asparagus, Broccoli, Bok Choy, Broccoli Rabe, Brussels Sprouts, Green Beans, Green Cabbage, Celery, Cucumbers, Endive, Leafy Greens (Examples: Kale, Mustard Greens), Leeks, Lettuce, Green Pepper, Snow Peas, Spinach, Watercress, Zucchini
❖	Purple	Purple cabbage, Eggplant

What About Organic?

Using organic foods will help to avoid the growing list of additives from artificial sweeteners to coloring agents that are finding their way into increasingly overly processed commercialized foods

You can go to www.foodnews.org to see a full list of fruits and vegetables and their ranking in terms of level of pesticides. Generally, when budget is a consideration, try to purchase organic for foods that are high in pesticides.

- ❖ Among the cleanest are onions, avocado, sweet corn (frozen), mango, kiwi fruit, asparagus, frozen sweet peas, cabbage, eggplant & broccoli.

- ❖ Those highest in pesticides are peaches, apples, lettuce, sweet bell peppers, celery, nectarines, strawberries, imported grapes, spinach and potatoes, imported blueberries, and kale

To claim that a product is "**100 percent Organic**" (or similar statement)

❖ The product must contain 100 percent organically produced ingredients, not counting added water and salt.

To claim that a food is "**Organic**" (or similar statement)

❖ The product must contain at least 95% organic ingredients, not counting added water and salt. Must not contain added sulfites.

❖ May contain up to 5% of: Non organically produced agricultural ingredients which are not commercially available in organic form; and/or other substances allowed by 7 CFR 205.605.

To claim that a product is "**Made with Organic Ingredients**" (or similar statement)

❖ The product must contain at least 70% organic ingredients, not counting added water and salt. The product must not contain added sulfites; except that, wine may contain added sulfur dioxide in accordance with 7 CFR 205.605.

❖ May contain up to 30% of: non organically produced agricultural ingredients; and/or other substances, including yeast, allowed by 7 CFR 205.605.

To claim that a product has some organic ingredients

❖ The product May contain less than 70% organic ingredients, not counting added water and salt.

❖ May contain over 30% of:Non-organically produced agricultural ingredients; and/or other substances, without being limited to those in 7 CFR 205.605

Starchy Vegetables

🔑 Starchy vegetables, like white potatoes, behave more like simple sugars. They break down quickly into glucose and causing a sharp insulin response and should be avoided. Other starchy vegetables such as yams and sweet potatoes cause a less dramatic insulin response and are excellent source of valuable nutrients.

❖ Yams, Sweet Potatoes	Substitute for White Potatoes. Yams and sweet potatoes cause a less dramatic insulin response and are excellent source of valuable nutrients
❖ Peas	Eat in moderation, great to keep on hand in freezer as compliment to salads and other dishes.
❖ Winter Squash	Eat in moderation
❖ Corn	Eat in moderation. Small amounts add flavor to tomato and bean salads.

Fruit

🔑 Avoid High Glycemic Fruit, including Melons (Honeydew, Cantaloupe, and Watermelon) Ripe Bananas, Pineapple, and Raisins.

❖ Blueberries	Low glycemic, excellent source of anti-oxidants
❖ Other Low-Medium Glycemic Fruit	Eat in moderation: Strawberries, raspberries, blackberries, boysenberries) , Lemon, Lime, Grapefruit, Peach, Apple, Plum, Pear, Peach, Orange, and Cherries

Whole grains

Eat sparingly depending upon your overall condition and blood sugar issues. Always combine cooked whole grains with vegetables and or protein and stay as close to the whole grain as possible. (Example: Steel cut oatmeal vs. more processed flakes)

❖ Gluten containing grains include wheat, barley, rye, and oats. Gluten free alternative flours include amaranth, buckwheat (not a wheat or grain, it is a plant in the same family as rhubarb), chestnut, corn, gram (from chickpeas) millet, quinoa, rice, soya and tapioca. Note: Oats do not contain gluten, but may be cross-contaminated during processing. There are companies that offer certified gluten free oatmeal.

❖ Quinoa	Low Glycemic, High in protein and fiber, gluten free
❖ Barley	Low Glycemic, avoid if gluten sensitive
❖ Buckwheat Groats	Low Glycemic (often referred to as "Kasha")
❖ Oatmeal	Steel Cut Oats, Oat Bran, Old Fashioned Oats (***always add protein***)
❖ Brown Rice	Higher on glycemic index, eat very sparingly

Bread, Crackers, Baked Goods

For optimum results, it is best to totally avoid or eat grain-based flour products. Grain-based flour based products have the same effect on blood sugar, whether the flour is produced from whole grains or not. Sprouted grain products are digested more like a vegetable with slower digestion and less of a spike in blood sugar. Sprouted grain breads will not have "flour" in the ingredients.

❖ If you have the time, your best bet for baked goods such as cookies or other treats is to make them yourself using non-grain based flour and sweetener of your choice.

❖ Breads: (purchase bread with 2-3+ Grams Fiber)	**Best breads**: Paleo Bread (Store bought or homemade), non-grain based flour breads (made with nut flour, bean flour, coconut flour. golden flax meal) Sprouted Whole Grain	Julian Bakery (Paleo products) Ezekiel 4:9™ Sprouted Grain Alvarado Street Bakery French Meadow Bakery Vermont Breads,.
❖ Cracker Substitutes	**Vegetable substitutes**: Zucchini or cucumber rounds, red/orange/yellow/green pepper slices, carrot/celery sticks	Sources for Occasional use: Wasa Crisp breads Mestemacher Three Grain Bread with Whole Rye Kernel Triscuits
❖ Non-grain based flour	**Nut flours** (almond, hazelnut, pecan, walnut) **Coconut flour** **Ground Flax Meal**	Paleo Baking Company Bob's Red Mill JK Gourmet Finely Ground Almond Flour

Pasta & Miscellaneous Grain Products

🔑 All pasta choices should be eaten sparingly, and mixed with vegetables and/or protein so that the pasta is more like a "condiment" to the other ingredients.

❖	Kashi 7 Whole Grain Nuggets	Use small amounts to make into "crunch" as topping for yogurt
❖	"No Sugar" Granola Mix	To use in nut mixes, to top yogurt or oatmeal
❖	Pasta	Sprouted Grain Pasta Buckwheat Soba Noodles

Legumes (fruits and seeds of leguminous plants)

🔑 Legumes are a good protein source and high in soluble fiber, but they also are high in phytic acid, which can affect mineral absorption. Proponents of certain diets, such as Paleo, say you should avoid all beans. But as long as you have a balanced food plan, eat beans in moderation and primarily eat beans that have been soaked before cooking, there is no need to avoid them totally and give up the benefits they provide.

❖	Soybeans	Keep frozen edamame on hand to toss into salads or to eat from the pods as a snack
❖	Adzuki Beans	Good for your kidneys, excellent in soup and stews
❖	Lentils	Red, Green, French (fast cooking, great for soups and quick salads)
❖	Red Kidney, Navy, White, Black Beans	All great for chili, stews, salads, salsas When using canned beans, rinse well to avoid consuming high levels of sodium
❖	Garbanzo Beans	Great for salads, making hummus, roasting as a snack

Meat. Poultry & Fish

🔑 If possible select organic meat & poultry products (no antibiotics, no added hormones, no animal by-products in feed and grass fed). Meat from grass fed animals contains more conjugated linoleic acid (a component of fat that boosts fat burning and the buildup of lean muscle mass) and more healthy Omega-3 fats. Organic sources will also be free of harmful hormone

❖	Poultry	Free Range Organic Chicken, Good Quality Turkey Breast
❖	Lean Meat	Lean cuts of beef or pork
❖	Fresh Fish	You can obtain a guide to ocean friendly seafood from the Blue Ocean Institute at www.blueocean.org . **Best**: High Eco Rating, low mercury content, high Omega 3 content **Examples**: Wild Salmon, Sardines, Herring, Sablefish, Albacore Tuna from U.S./Canada, Farm Raised Oysters.
❖	Tofu	Firm, Soft(good for puddings & sauces) (don't overdo eating processed soy and look for non-GMO brands)
❖	Canned Sardines	Crown Prince (has boneless variety if preferred)

Healthy Fats & Oils

Try to limit amount of Oils to 1-2 Tablespoons daily & get the rest of your fats from food sources. Eat no more than ¼ cup of nuts & seeds daily.

- ❖ *Monounsaturated Fats*: Sources include: Olive Oil, Canola Oil, Avocados, Almonds
- ❖ *Omega-3 Fats*: Sources include: flaxseeds & flaxseed oil, walnuts & walnut oil, salmon, herring, fresh tuna, sardines, pumpkin seeds. Depending on your health goals and condition, you may want to supplement your diet with a high quality fish oil.

❖ Extra Virgin Olive Oil	Organic if possible. (Bionaturae Organic Extra Virgin Olive Oil).
❖ Avocados	Slice on salads, use in dips & salad dressing, enjoy Guacamole
❖ Other Oils	Coconut oil, Walnut Oil, Sesame Oil, Canola Oil (Use Sparingly)

Nuts & Seeds

❖ Seeds	Pumpkin, Sunflower, Sesame Seeds, Chia
❖ Assorted Nuts	Almonds, Walnuts, Pecans, Pistachio Nuts, Brazil Nuts
❖ Flax Seeds	**Whole**-Use coffee grinder to grind small portions at a time **Ground**- Bob's Red Mill, Barleans (keep refrigerated)

Eggs, Dairy, Dairy Substitutes

❖ Low Fat Milk	Over the Moon (is a more full bodied brand of skim milk)
❖ Low Fat Ricotta	Good to have on hand for spreads, dips, puddings and sugar free dessert alternatives
❖ Milk Alternatives	Rice, Coconut, Almond milk etc. (look for unsweetened brands)
❖ Butter or Butter Alternatives	NO TRANSFATS
❖ Eggs/Egg Whites	Enriched with Omega 3, Organic, Free Range
❖ Plain Yogurt	Flavor with stevia, sugar free jams, fruit etc.(Greek Yogurt is lower in lactose and has twice the protein content of regular yogurt)
❖ Low Fat Cheese	Goat Cheese, Laughing Cow Wedges, String Cheese

Vinegar, Salad Dressings, Marinades, Liquid Seasonings

❖ Vinegars	Red Wine, Balsamic , Apple Cider (Braggs), Rice (Nakano-no sugar)
❖ Mirin	A type of Rice Cooking Wine-(Eden Foods\- no sugar added)
❖ Braggs Liquid Amino Acids	Use in place of soy sauce
❖ Salad Dressings (no Sugar Added)	Newman's Own Olive Oil & Vinegar; Trader Joes Red Wine & Olive Oil Vinaigrette; Annies Tuscany Italian Dressing; Annies Goddess Dressing
❖ Marinades, Sauces	Drew's dressings & marinades; (look for varieties with no added sugars), Worcestershire Sauce

Condiments, Seasonings & Miscellaneous

❖	Seasonings	Cinnamon, Vanilla, Garlic, Ginger, Tumeric, Pepper, Fine Herbs, Cilantro, Chili Powder, Paprika, Garam Masala
❖	Gomashio	This is a mixture of ground sesame seeds and sea salt. Excellent on greens & grains
❖	Seasoning Mixes	Trader Joe's 21 Salute, other low salt, sugar free mixes Bittersweet Herb Farm, Penzys
❖	Protein Powder	Jay Robb, PGX Satisfast (look for brands without added sugar)
❖	Sugar Free Jams/Jelly	Look for Organic, Blueberry/Strawberry
❖	Almond Butter	Raw or Roasted.
❖	Sugar Alternatives	Stevia, Xylitol, Erythritol. Stevia is available on line at www.sweetleaf.com and at many food stores in liquid and powder form. Liquid Stevia is available in various flavors..
❖	Unsweetened Cocoa or Raw Cacao	Chocolate is full of healthy antioxidants. (learn more about raw chocolate at www.sunfood.com)
❖	Cacao Nibs	Raw cacao nibs can be added to oatmeal, used in desserts, or eaten on their own with a little agave syrup.
❖	Dark Chocolate	Lily's or Coco Polo Dark Chocolate, (Sweetened with Stevia & Erythritol)
❖	Tea	Green Tea (various flavors); Roobis Tea, herbal teas
❖	Coffee Alternatives	Teeccino; Ganocafe
❖	Soup Stock	Organic Chicken, Vegetable Broth
❖	Canned Tomatoes	Pomi, Muir Glen, or other all natural, low sodium brand
❖	Marinara/Pasta Sauce	Choose brands that do not have any added sugar
❖	Mustard	Dijon, Pommery
❖	Salsa & Hot Sauce	Salsa: No added sugar brand such as Newman's Own Hot Sauce: Tabasco or another all natural hot sauce
❖	Pickles & Sauerkraut	You can get raw sauerkraut from Rejuvenative Foods or Glaser Organic Farms. Bubbies is also a good brand.
❖	Canned Soups & Chili	Health Valley, Amy's Kitchen (Look for low sodium & no added sugars)
❖	Bagged Beans	Good as soup starters
❖	Seltzer	Plain & flavored
❖	Hummus	Cedars, Sabra
❖	Bean & Tofu Dips	Michelle's Tofu Tahini Dip
❖	Sun Dried Tomatoes	Organic Sundried Tomatoes (Mediterranean Organics®)
❖	Capers	Organic Wild Capers (Mediterranean Organics®)
❖	Light Mayonnaise	(Some brands now have Olive Oil in their ingredients)
❖	Nori Sea Vegetable	Eat as a snack or use to make nori sushi rolls. (seasnax®)

Janet's Pantry

People always ask me what my "must have" pantry items are. So here is a list of my favorite things and food items that I always keep on hand.

- ❖ **Non-Starchy Vegetables**
  - Yams/Sweet Potatoes
  - Frozen Peas & Frozen Corn
- ❖ **Vegetables (shop for other veggies daily)**
  - Carrots
  - Cucumbers
  - Frozen Edamame
  - Fresh & Minced Garlic , Fresh Ginger
  - Green & Red Cabbage
  - Kale, Celery, Romaine Lettuce (for green drink)
  - Lettuce mixes
  - Onions,
  - Peppers (red, yellow, green)
  - Tomatoes
  - Mushrooms (fresh and dried)
- ❖ **Fruit** – These are the fruits I always have available.
  - Acai Berry (Powder & Frozen)
  - Blueberries (Frozen & Fresh in summer)
  - Citrus Fruits (Lemons, Limes, Grapefruit)
- ❖ **Whole Grains**
  - Barley
  - Quinoa (Red & White)
  - Steel Cut Oats
- ❖ **Nuts, Seeds & Nut Butters**
  - Almonds, Pecans, Walnuts
  - Raw Pumpkin Seeds
  - Roasted Sunflower Seeds
  - Ground Flax Seeds (Barleans), Ground Flax Meal for baking (Bob's Red Mill),
  - Chia Seeds
  - Almond Butter (Raw & Regular), Peanut Butter
  - Tahini
- ❖ **Beans**
  - Canned: Garbanzo, Black, Navy
  - Dried: Lentils, Adzuki Beans
  - Amy's Chili
  - Bagged Bean Mixes
  - Hummus & Other Bean Spreads
- ❖ **Marinades & Stir Fry Seasonings**
  - Drew's Dressing & Marinades (No sugar added)
  - Bragg's Liquid Amino Acids
  - Ponzu Sauce (no sugar added)
- ❖ **Healthy Fats & Oils**
  - Olive Oil (Extra Virgin and flavored)
  - Avocados
  - Coconut Oil, Walnut Oil
- ❖ **Seasonings**
  - Cinnamon, Vanilla,, Tumeric, Pepper, Fine Herbs, Basil, Cilantro, Chili Powder, Paprika, Parsley, Garam Masala, Gomashio, Mexican blend, Garlic powder, Sea Salt, Trader Joe's 21 Salute

- ❖ **Breads , Cereal, Pasta, Crackers & Chips**
  - Sprouted Grain Bread, English Muffins & Tortillas
  - Rolled Oats (for baking & Granola)
  - Soba Noodles, Whole Wheat Penne
  - Paleo Bread/Wraps
  - Nut flours, (Almond, Hazelnut), Coconut flour for baking
  - Baking Soda, Baking Powder
  - Stevia in the Raw (for Baking)
- ❖ **Vinegar, Salad Dressings, Marinades**
  - Vinegars: Red Wine, Balsamic, Rice, Ume Plum, Citrus Flavored, Apple Cider Vinegar
  - Salad Dressings: Newman's Own Olive Oil & Vinegar, Annie's Goddess, Trader Joe's Olive Oil and Red Wine
- ❖ **Dairy, Protein & Milk Alternatives** (In addition to items below, I buy fish, meat, poultry as needed)
  - Goat Cheese (spreadable & regular)
  - Greek Yogurt (Fage)
  - Laughing Cow Cheese Wedges
  - Fresh Parmesan Cheese
  - Part Skim Ricotta
  - Tofu (Firm & Silky)
  - Butter (Grass Fed)
  - Almond Milk - Unsweetened
  - Coconut Milk - Unsweetened
  - Organic Cooked Roasted Chicken
  - Sardines (Crown Prince Boneless)
  - Free Range, Organic Eggs
- ❖ **Condiments, & Miscellaneous**
  - Mustard,
  - Light Mayonnaise
  - Sun Dried Tomatoes,
  - Capers
  - Fresh Garlic and Ginger
  - Greens Powder, Whey Protein Powder Satisfast/PGX Whey Protein Mix
  - Organic Soup Stock (Chicken and Vegetable)
  - Worcestershire Sauce
  - Salsa
  - Unsweetened Raw Cacao
  - Goji Powder (for smoothies)
  - Dark Chocolate (Lillys, Coco Polo)
  - Tea (Green & Black)
  - Seltzer & Sparkling Water
  - Tomato Sauce/Pasta Sauce/Pizza Sauce
  - Stevia (Powder and Liquid:
  - Fruit Spreads (Wild Blueberry)
  - Nori Sea Vegetable for nori rolls and for snacking

Meal Planning

Over the course of the day, your food intake should "approximate" the percentages shown in the diagram below.

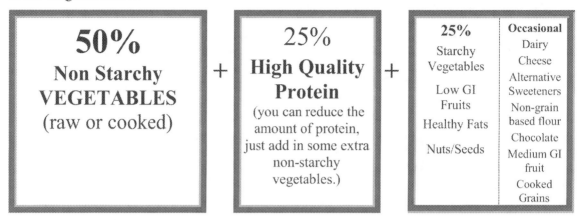

Ideally 75% of what you eat on a daily basis will consist of non-starchy vegetables and high quality protein. But, for long term success, remember that eating is not a science.

Each day strive to get as close to the LIVE FREE Food Plan as possible, based on the food suggestions set forth in this workbook. BUT, you don't have to be exact and you don't have to give up enjoying all your favorite foods or follow a food plan of deprivation.

So, if for example, you have a day where you ate mostly starchy vegetables, fruit, cheese and sprouted grain bread or even some grain-based flour-products, that is OK. The key is that if you find yourself getting into that that pattern over several days, it is time to recommit to the LIVE FREE food plan basics and get back on track.

Another way to look at menu planning is to visualize what your plate might look like at each meal as shown in the diagram below. It is deliberately a simple plan. There is no need to count or measure. Just keep at close as you can to the percentages, watch portion sizes and be extra vigilant with foods in the "Eat Sparingly" and "Totally Avoid" categories. If you are planning a one pot meal such as a stew or with multiple ingredients such as a stir fry, estimate the percentages of the ingredients and add a salad for good measure.

*NOTE:"*Other*" foods in the diagram below should include those from the **25% and Occasional** block shown above. Breakfast is one meal where you might not consume as many vegetables, but try to include a hearty portion at least 3-5 times per week.

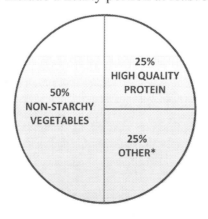

Here is a Recap of the foods to choose in the LIVE FREE Food Plan™.

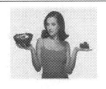

As you being to adopt new habits and follow the food plan on a daily basis, your body will respond and it will become a way of life that comes naturally to you. And that is the secret to long term change.

You will find over time that even "splurges" start to look and feel different when you choose treats from the "Enjoy Occasionally" and "Eat Sparingly" group rather than those foods in the "Totally Avoid" columns..

EAT MORE:

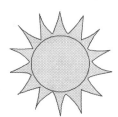

Non-Starchy Vegetables – 50%

- Cooked or Raw
- Green/Veggie Smoothies
- Green/Veggie Juices

NOTE: You can eat less protein, just add some extra non-starchy vegetables

HEALTHY PROTEIN – 25%

- Lean/Grass Fed Beef, Organic/Free Range Poultry, Lean Pork
- Fish (Best: High Eco Rating, low mercury content, high Omega 3 content)
    Examples: Wild Salmon, Sardines, Herring, Sablefish, Albacore Tuna from U.S./Canada, Farm Raised Oysters)
- Legumes (Soaked, maximum- one serving daily)
- Tofu, Tempeh (avoid highly processed soy products)
- Eggs, Yogurt, Kefir

DON'T OVER EAT these nutrient rich foods:

Small Portions - 25%

Starchy Vegetables
Low GI Fruits
Healthy Fats -Nuts/Seeds

ENJOY Occasionally

Dark Chocolate (Sweetened with Stevia or 70-80% Cocoa)
Baked Goods made with sprouted grains or Non-Grain Based Flour (Nut, Seed, Bean, Coconut)
Stevia

EAT SPARINGLY

Medium/High GI Fruits	Fish with low eco-rating, high mercury, low omega 3 content (Example: Farm Raised Salmon)	Dairy (chesse, milk, sour cream, cottage cheese, cream chease)	Coffee
Cooked Whole Grains			
Sugar Alternatives (Sugar Alcohols, Splenda, etc.)	Highly Processed Soy Products	Saturated Fats (butter, any fat that turns solid)	

Totally Avoid

Grain Based Flour Simple Sugars Aspartame High fructose corn syrup.	High fat/ sodium processed meats	Trans Fats	Soda (Regular or Diet)
	Fish high in contaminants		

Cooking with The Crave Control Kitchen™ and Coach N' Cook Free-form Recipes

CRAVECONTROLKITCHEN™

CONQUER CRAVINGS WITH OUR TIPS, TRICKS & RECIPES

If the word "cooking" conjures up pulling out a recipe, scrambling to get the "correct" ingredients, and hours spent preparing foods from scratch you are among the millions who would rather dine out or do "take out" any day.

Cooking real food for yourself and your loved ones will transform your health and is the true foundation of blood sugar health. So if you find yourself constantly craving foods that don't serve your well-being, but you "hate to cook", the next sections are for you.

First, let's talk about recipes.

I am the first to admit that I am a big fan of recipe books. I have over 100 in my collection, and I love reading them and exploring new ideas. So it might surprise you if I said that when it comes to day-to-day cooking, I very rarely use a recipe for anything other than inspiration for a dish based on what is in my refrigerator, freezer and pantry.

For years I have been cooking using what I call a "Free Form Recipe" approach. Today, this approach is trending, and some cooks call this style of cooking improvisational cooking or recipe-less cooking. It is a fluid type of food preparation that will enable you to prepare satisfying and delicious meals more spontaneously with what you have on hand..

The common denominator for this type of food preparation is the idea that recipes are guides based upon a "formula" for a particular type of food. Once you know the basic formula underlying a recipe you can swap out ingredients and change amounts based on what is available as well as your own tastes and preferences.

Crave Control Kitchen Coach N' Cook recipes have both a coaching component where I explain the ingredients and basic formula for a preparing a dish along with preparation techniques, and then I set forth a basic free-form recipe with some suggestions for swapping out ingredients. The key is to understand basic techniques and how recipes work, and then the possibilities are endless. The essential recipes are simple and require only a few ingredients. You can embellish and add from there based on your taste and creativity.

Final Thoughts:

Measurements: in some of my free form recipes I include basic measurements so that you have an idea where to start. In most cases it is more than OK to vary the amount based on taste and how many people you are preparing food for. (The one exception is baking, where measurements generally should be followed for optimum results) If you are not sure how much of an ingredient or seasoning to add, the best technique is to add a little at a time. A little common sense comes in handy here. I very often do a taste test as I go along.

But NOT, if I am preparing certain raw food. So, I might taste a spoonful of mashed sweet potatoes to see if I have added enough cinnamon, and I might taste a marinade BEFORE pouring over raw chicken. But I am not going to taste ingredients once they are poured onto raw poultry until it has been cooked thoroughly. At the end, before serving I might taste to see if anything extra is needed.

Ingredients: It is always OK to swap out ingredients. (Baking is usually an exception, *unless* the recipe provides alternative ingredients) For example if you are making a stir fry that calls for string beans and you don't have any, use broccoli, it will be fine. If you find a great smoothie recipe that includes peanut butter and you only have almond butter on hand, use that instead. Don't want to thicken your smoothie with sugar laden bananas? I have a smoothie for breakfast every day, and I haven't had a banana in years. If I find a recipe with banana that looks good, I substitute ice and or chia for the thickener and stevia for sweetness. Have a great French Toast recipe? Swap out the grain-based flour bread and use a Paleo or sprouted grain bread instead.

Cooking "from Scratch": With so many options available today ranging from salad bars to fancy in store deli's and other pre-made foods, cooking a delicious and healthy meal doesn't necessarily mean that every ingredient has be made from scratch. Roasted chicken is a great example. Many stores offer prepared free range roasted chicken that can be used in a variety of ways.

For example I often shred the meat from the breasts to make Chinese Chicken salad. Then I use the bones and dark meat to make a hearty chicken soup. Or you can save time chopping and cutting by buying pre-cut vegetables and salad greens. Canned goods are also a great way to get a meal together quickly. Amy's makes a good chili that becomes delicious when you add your own seasonings, sautéed onions and carrots. Feel like some meat? Add grass-fed lean ground beef. The possibilities are endless.

Using detailed recipes: There are going to be times when you want a specific recipe. (such as for entertaining or baking). For these occasions, I definitely recommend having a few cookbooks on hand, or if you prefer you can go on-line to the hundreds of available cooking sites.

Now, let's take a look at an example Coach N' Cook free-form recipe, **Yogurt Breakfast Parfait**.

There are hundreds of recipes in food magazines, cookbooks and on-line for what is essentially yogurt layered with fruit and a garnish.

The Yogurt Parfait recipe below combines creamy yogurt, antioxidant rich blueberries & strawberries, and satisfying "cereal crunch", to make a Yogurt Parfait that is quick, delicious and versatile.

It is great for a quick breakfast, as a snack, and you can even serve it as an elegant dessert. Try sprinkling some dark chocolate bits or shavings on top for an added touch of elegance & sweetness. (and added antioxidants!)

So what if dessert is actually "healthy", your family or guests will love it and they won't suspect a thing.

Basic Yogurt Parfait Formula:

[Yogurt + Sweetener of Choice + Flavoring of Choice] + Layered Fruit + Garnish/Crunch

Ingredients:

- ❖ **Plain Yogurt**: One cup of yogurt will yield 2 small parfaits. I suggest using Greek Yogurt. (My favorite is Fage)

- ❖ **Sweetener of Choice**: The amount varies depending on how sweet you want the result to be Suggested options: Small amount of agave syrup and Stevia (combined); Vanilla Sugar Free Syrup by DaVinci or Torani. Walden Farms Sugar Free Maple Syrup, Coconut Nectar, Liquid or powered Stevia.

- ❖ **Cinnamon**: In this recipe I use cinnamon to flavor the yogurt. I like to add cinnamon because it adds to the overall sweetness in the taste of the yogurt and it also helps to regulate blood sugars. For a whole different feel, you could add some raw cacao or other cocoa powder. But remember that cocoa is more bitter so when you add cocoa you usually need to add a little more sweetener.

- ❖ **Fruit**: I generally use fresh or frozen blueberries and/or cut up strawberries: You need about a cup of fruit for 2 parfaits. You can really use any fruit, but my suggestion for the optimum health benefit is to use low glycemic fruits such as berries, kiwi, peaches and avoid high glycemic fruits such as melons, grapes and ripe bananas.

- ❖ **"Crunch"**: Below is a "crunch" I make using Ezekial 4:9 Almond Sprouted Whole Grain Cereal. It is very easy to make and adds a healthy crunch to the parfait. If you don't want to get involved in making the crunch, you can substitute a fruit sweetened granola. Or you can use a combination of roasted or raw nuts such as walnuts or pecans. Your favorite trail mix is also a good option.

How to Make the Parfait:

- ❖ **Prepare the Crunch**: Heat up a heavy skillet, and add 1/4 to 1/2 box of Ezekial 4:9 Almond Sprouted Whole Grain Cereal to the warm skillet. Sprinkle some cinnamon over the cereal, and pour small amount of sweetener of choice over the cereal to sweeten it. (I use granulated Stevia and a very small amount of Agave) Then mix the cinnamon and sweetener into the cereal, stirring it for about 5 minutes over low heat to blend it all into the cereal and to slightly roast the cereal mixture. Remove from heat, and put in bowl to cool. Depending on the sweetener used, the mixture may stick together when it cools down--use a fork to gently break it apart.

- ❖ **Prepare the Yogurt**: Place the yogurt in a bowl and add a small amount of sweetener and cinnamon. Mix the sweetener and cinnamon into the yogurt. Taste, and add more sweetener and cinnamon if needed.

- ❖ **Prepare The Fruit**: Wash & rinse the fruit. Cut the strawberries into small pieces.

- ❖ **Assemble the Parfaits**: Place a tablespoon of the crunch in the bottom of the glasses or parfait glasses. Next, place approximately 1/4 cup of the yogurt on top of the crunch. Top with 1/4 cup of the sliced strawberries. Repeat the layers. Optional: Top with shaved dark chocolate.

GREENS:

Leafy green vegetables are high in calcium, magnesium, iron potassium, phosphorous, zinc, and vitamins A, C, E, and K. They are also great sources of fiber, folic acid, chlorophyll, and many other micronutrients and phytochemicals.

Kale, in particular, is a powerhouse vegetable, and in fact, is one of the highest ranking vegetables on the ORAC scale. This is a rating that is based upon a method of measuring the antioxidant capacity of fruits and vegetables. Foods are ranked according to their potential to mop up oxygen free radicals. Choosing foods with a high ORAC value gives you an extra boost. The top 10 ORAC scores per 4 oz. fresh produce include: blueberries, blackberries, garlic, kale, strawberries, spinach, Brussels sprouts, alfalfa sprouts, and broccoli.

Kale contains seven times the beta carotene of broccoli and ten times as much lutein and zeaxanthin. These are eye protecting carotenoids that are known to protect against macular degeneration. Most people are familiar with garden variety greens such as spinach and romaine lettuce, but shy away from other varieties of greens such as arugula, kale, bok choy, collards and mustard greens.

Serving Suggestions:

❖ Make a salad of arugula, red onion, pine nuts and shaved parmesan cheese tossed with a light vinaigrette (olive oil/balsamic vinegar)

❖ Lightly boil some kale, chop it up finely and add it to some cooked grains. (such as barley or quinoa) For variety add other chopped vegetables or sun-dried tomatoes.

❖ Add some cooked chopped kale to your regular salad.

❖ Add some kale to winter soups such as minestrone

❖ Lightly sauté some kale in olive oil. Add pine nuts and minced garlic for extra flavor.

❖ Lightly boil kale. Chop finely and sprinkle with rice vinegar. For extra flavor sprinkle on some Gomashio. (a seasoning made of ground sesame seeds and other spices)

❖ Mix chopped kale with finely chopped sauerkraut, coleslaw, or pressed red cabbage.

Basic "Quick" Boiled Kale:

3/4 lbs. kale

2 cups water

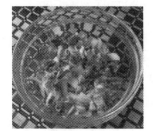

❖ Wash kale well, checking on the underside of leaves for any grey/green aphids which sometimes cling to kale leaves.

❖ Either use your hands to strip the kale leaves off the stalk or use a knife to cut the leaves from the stalk. (you can cook the stalk in the boiling water separately and chop. The stalks take a little longer to cook)

❖ Chop or tear the kale into medium size pieces

❖ Bring the water to a boil.

❖ Add the kale to the water and bring it back to a boil. Allow the kale to remain in the water until it turns a bright green color. (3-4 minutes) *Do Not Overcook*

❖ Remove the kale from the water with a slotted spoon. Then, chop the kale into small pieces and use it in any of the recipes above.

How to Make A Super Salad: Greens + Dressing + Veggies/Protein + Condiments

❖ **Use a variety of greens**: There are many delicious and highly nutritious varieties of leafy greens available as an alternative to traditional iceberg lettuce. Try Arugula, Butterhead lettuce, Curly Endive, Mache, Mesclun, Romaine, Spinach, Watercress or Kale for a flavorful salad that is rich in nutrients.

❖ **Add a variety of healthy vegetables and/or protein and condiments**: Adding vegetables and/or protein and condiments such as nuts or seeds or cheese such as shaved parmesan or goat cheese makes your salad even more nutritious and provides a delicious balance of flavors and colors. Here are some ideas:

▪ **GREEN**: Boston lettuce, Baby Spinach, Romaine, Watercress, Parsley, Mixed Field Greens, Arugula, Green Peppers, Chopped Kale, Pumpkin Seeds, Green Cabbage, Broccoli, Celery, Cucumber, Sprouts, Green Olives, Avocado.

▪ **YELLOW/ORANGE**: Yellow Bell Pepper, Dried Apricot, Carrots, Mango, Sliced Orange, Small amounts of corn as a garnish, Pinto Beans.

▪ **BLUE/PURPLE**: Blueberries, Red Grapes, Eggplant, Mission Figs, Blackberries, Arame (a type of sea vegetable often used as a salad ingredient in Japanese cuisine)

▪ **WHITE**: Reduced Fat Goat Cheese, Jicama, Cauliflower, Firm Tofu, Mushrooms, Sunflower Seeds, Sesame Seeds, Garlic, Pine Nuts

▪ **RED**: Tomatoes, Red Kidney Beans, Red Bell Pepper, Red Onion, Radicchio, Red Cabbage, Red Apple Slices, Red Onions, Sun Dried Tomatoes

❖ **Choose healthy oils for your salad dressings**: Extra Virgin Olive oil is a good choice. Try this simple recipe for a light, refreshing dressing:

▪ 1 tsp olive oil, ¼ cup lemon juice/ or lime juice, 2 tbs. chopped fresh parsley, 2 tbs. finely chopped onion, 1 clove garlic- finely chopped. Combine all ingredients and mix thoroughly. Add salt and pepper to taste.

▪ When buying ready-made dressings, choose dressings made with Olive Oil and little or no sugar. A good brand is Newman's Own. You can add a little Apple Cider vinegar or Red Wine vinegar to give the dressing extra flavor.

▪ Another fool proof way to "dress" your salad is to drizzle a small amount of extra virgin olive oil on the greens and mix in well. The greens should be lightly dressed, not soggy. Then add a small amount of vinegar of choice or lemon juice to taste. Finally, add any seasonings and your veggies/protein and/or condiments.

Easy Tomato, Avocado Salad with Tuna

Looking for a quick lunch that is filling and easy to prepare?
A tomato salad can be a springboard for a variety of salads depending on what you have on hand. For a basic tomato salad, cut 10-12 cherry tomatoes in half. Place in a bowl with ½ avocado, cut into small pieces. Squeeze fresh lime juice over the tomatoes and avocado. Season with a dash of sea salt or Braggs Liquid Aminos. Top with a scoop of Tuna Salad.

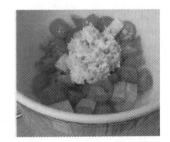

For a more complex salad, add any of the following: corn, black beans, chopped red onion or cucumber. Experiment with different dressings.

QUINOA:

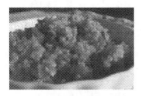 Quinoa has an exceptionally high nutritional profile and cooks the fastest of all grains. When it is cooked, the outer germ surrounding the seed breaks open to form a crunchy coil while the inner part of the grain becomes soft and translucent. It is a very versatile grain that is as delicious as a hearty salad with vegetables and condiments as it is when served as a breakfast porridge with nuts and fruit.

Nutritional Highlights

❖ Quinoa contains all eight amino acids to make it a complete protein.

❖ Quinoa is high in B vitamins, iron, zinc, potassium, calcium and vitamin E.

❖ Quinoa is gluten free and easy to digest. It is strengthening for the kidneys, heart and lungs.

Preparation:

❖ Rinse one cup of quinoa well with cool water in a fine mesh strainer until the water runs clear. [**ALWAYS** rinse quinoa before cooking to thoroughly remove the bitter coating, called saponin. Saponin is a naturally occurring toxin that coats the quinoa grain. Quinoa is rinsed before packaging, to remove the saponin, but it is best to rinse again before cooking.]

❖ Combine the quinoa and 2 cups water in a saucepan. Cover and bring to a boil. (for extra flavor try chicken or vegetable broth in place of water)

❖ Reduce the heat to a simmer and continue to cook covered for about 15 minutes or until all the water has been absorbed.

❖ Remove from the heat and let stand for 5 minutes covered, then fluff with a fork.

Quinoa Salad Ideas:

Cooked Quinoa + Chopped Vegetables + Dressing + Seasoning + Protein and/or Garnish

❖ **Prepare Quinoa** – Per instructions above

❖ **Prepare Vegetables:** Dice 2-4 vegetables of choice. For more intense flavor, you can marinate one or more of the vegetables before adding them to the cooked Quinoa. For example, you can marinate chopped red onions in balsamic vinegar.

❖ **Add Dressing:** Drizzle a very small amount of olive oil over the quinoa mixture and lightly toss to coat the quinoa. Then add a clear vinegar, such as rice vinegar, champagne or citrus flavored vinegar to taste. (for a very light salad, you can omit the olive oil).

❖ **Add Seasonings:** Add seasonings of choice and lightly toss to mix.

❖ **Add Garnish:** Add garnishes such as pumpkin or sunflower seeds for crunch.

❖ **Add Protein Choice:** If desired add beans, tofu, chicken or salmon for a heartier salad.

Try one of the combinations below with cooked quinoa or invent a combo of your own

❖ Diced (red onion, tomato, red or green pepper) and lightly steamed corn removed from cob

❖ Quartered cherry tomato, diced (cucumber, green or red pepper, and carrot) with chopped parsley (For Traditional Tabouleh salad-add olive oil & lemon dressing with a touch of garlic)

❖ Diced marinated red onion, chopped sundried tomato, lightly steamed, chopped kale. Garnish with sunflower or pumpkin seeds. Steamed Corn is great with this combo as well.

❖ Diced marinated red onion, petite peas, water chestnuts Garnish with chopped pecans.

Other Serving Suggestions

- **Emerald Quinoa:** Prepare Quinoa. While quinoa is cooking, sauté diced onion until soft and sweet tasting. Set onions aside. Lightly boil some kale, chop it up finely. Lightly boil some Broccoli crowns and cut them into small pieces. Put ¼ cup frozen peas in a strainer and run under very hot water for 3-4 minutes until thawed. Mix the onions and all of the vegetables in with the quinoa. Season with Gomashio and your choice of: Braggs Liquid Amino Acids, Ponzu Sauce (an Asian seasoning that is a combination of Rice Vinegar, Mirin and Tamari) or Tamari Soy Sauce. (use the liquid sparingly and season to taste)

- **Super Quick Quinoa with Peas, Onions & Chopped Arugula**: Prepare Quinoa per directions. Lightly sauté diced onion and in small amount of olive or sesame oil in a medium sized skillet. Defrost ½ cup of frozen peas by placing in strainer and running under hot water for 2-3 minutes. Add the quinoa and peas to the onions. Sauté lightly for 2-3 minutes. Add chopped arugula. Sauté for another minute. Season to taste. Garnish with Nuts or Seeds of choice. (if desired add some canned beans or leftover fish/chicken)..

- **Quinoa with Sundried Tomatoes, Onions & Corn:** Cook Quinoa. While quinoa is cooking, sauté diced onion until soft and sweet tasting. Lightly steam 2 ears of corn and remove corn from the cob. Dice enough sundried tomatoes to measure ¼ cup. Add all ingredients to the Quinoa. Season to taste with an all-purpose seasoning blend such as Trader Joes 21 Salute, Braggs Liquid Amino Acids or Tamari Soy Sauce.

- **Quinoa with Pressed Red Cabbage**: Cook Quinoa. (try using Tri-Colored Quinoa which nicely complements the red cabbage). Slice 1/4-1/2 red cabbage lengthwise. (i.e. shred the cabbage as you would to make coleslaw) Next, follow the directions for *Easy Pressed Cabbage* set forth at the bottom of the following page. Once the cabbage is pressed, dice enough cabbage to equal 1 cup and add the diced pressed cabbage to the quinoa. If desired sprinkle with Gomashio to taste. Variations: Add some chopped apple, parsley and walnuts for a Quinoa Waldorf Salad. Instead of lemon, squeeze the juice of an orange to add a zesty citrus flavor to the salad.

- **Quinoa with Black Bean Salsa**: Cook Quinoa. Set aside. Rinse contents of one can of black beans. Mix beans with diced red and orange bell peppers, chopped tomato, and chopped red onion. Drizzle small amount of olive oil over beans and mix well. Add rice vinegar to taste. If desired add some chopped cilantro and/or sprinkle with some lime juice. Add bean mixture to the quinoa.

- **Breakfast Quinoa Porridge**: To prepare cook the quinoa following the regular preparation directions. If time is an issue, you can cook the quinoa the night before and store it in the refrigerator. To prepare a serving of cereal, place a cup of quinoa in a saucepan. Add a splash of milk (skim or low fat) or soy or other nut milk to the cooked quinoa and heat through stirring to make the mixture slightly creamy. You can add one or more of the following for variety and added health benefits: cinnamon, ground flax seeds, whey powder, wheat germ, blueberries, roasted yams or squash, chopped nuts (walnuts, almonds, or pecans).

BROCCOLI & CRUCIFEROUS VEGETABLES

Broccoli is a member of the Brassica family of cruciferous vegetables. These vegetables are excellent sources of anticancer phytochemicals called isothiocyantes. Isothiocyantes fight cancer by neutralizing carcinogens in our bodies. In addition broccoli is a great source of the vitamin C, folate, potassium, fiber, vitamin E and vitamin B6 all of which promote cardiovascular health. Broccoli is also a bone builder. One cup of raw broccoli provides 41 milligrams of calcium along with 79 milligrams of vitamin C which promotes the absorption of calcium. Broccoli also provides vitamin K, which is important for blood clotting and also contributes to bone health. **Other cruciferous vegetables** that are high in nutrients include: Brussels sprouts, kale, cabbage, cauliflower, collards, bok choy, mustard greens, arugula, watercress, daikon root, and swiss chard.

Serving Suggestions:

- ❖ Puree leftover broccoli with some sautéed onions and mix with low-fat milk or almond milk with seasonings (try nutmeg) for a fast creamy soup
- ❖ Lightly steam or quick boil some broccoli and eat with low fat dip dressing
- ❖ Stir fry shredded cabbage (add onions for extra flavor)
- ❖ Roast broccoli, cauliflower with olive oil and a touch of balsamic vinegar
- ❖ Sauté very small pieces of chopped cauliflower as a substitute for rice. (don't overcook)
- ❖ Server raw or lightly steamed broccoli florets with hummus dip
- ❖ Sprinkle lemon juice and sesame seeds over lightly steamed broccoli
- ❖ Combine steamed quartered Brussels sprouts with sliced red onions, walnuts, and some mild tasting cheese (such as feta). Toss with olive oil and balsamic vinegar for a light side dish.
- ❖ Sauté broccoli with red peppers, garlic and olive oil. (Dress with small of lemon)

Easy Pressed Red Cabbage:

Sliced Cabbage + Salt + Press + Rinse + Season + (Other Veggies /Condiments)

Red or purple cabbage is also a source of anthocyanins, pigment molecules that make blueberries blue and red cabbage red. The ability of Anthocyanins to act as antioxidants to fight free radical make them powerful weapons against cardiovascular disease, and they are also known for their anti-inflammatory effect. In addition to the many nutritional benefits of cabbage, it is a great source of fiber. One cup of cooked cabbage gives you almost 4 grams of fiber. The recipe below is a very basic cabbage salad. You can dress it up by adding seeds, apples, or other shredded vegetables.

Ingredients:

½ small head green cabbage

1 tsp sea salt

2 tsp vinegar of choice or lemon juice

1 tsp olive oil

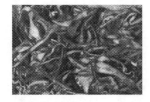

Slice the cabbage lengthwise.

Put in bowl and sprinkle with enough salt to draw water from the cabbage. Mix well. Place a plate on top of the cabbage and weigh it down with something heavy that will press the plate down. Allow the cabbage to sit in the bowl for approximately ½ hour to 1 hour. (the salt removes water and acid from the cabbage)

Next, squeeze the cabbage gently between your hands to release the water, or if desired, rinse cabbage lightly to remove most of the salt. Then drain & squeeze well. Combine the olive oil and vinegar or olive oil with lemon juice and pour over the cabbage & toss. (you can omit the olive oil for a lighter dressing)

SWEET POTATOES

Sweet potatoes are high in fiber and nutrients and are a better choice than white potatoes which have a more dramatic effect on blood sugars. Sweet potatoes are a rich source of antioxidants, especially beta-carotene, vitamin A, and potassium. They also contain health promoting phytochemicals, such as quercetin, a powerful anti-inflammatory, and chlorogenic acid, an antioxidant.

I find that sweet potatoes, in moderation, are a satisfying substitute for sugar laden foods, and that including them in my food plan helps to cut back on sugar cravings. The great thing about sweet potatoes is that they are so versatile and can be prepared in a number of ways. Below are some ideas for preparing sweet potatoes. (For any of the recipe ideas you can either remove the skins or keep them on which will increase the amount of fiber.)

- ❖ Bake a sweet potato and enjoy it with a small amount of healthy butter alternative and a dash of agave syrup
- ❖ Cut up 1-2 sweet potatoes into cubed pieces & roast. (see Recipes on following page).
- ❖ Add sautéed onions and peppers to roasted sweet potato cubes for a healthier version of sweet potato hash browns
- ❖ Add roasted sweet potato cubes to oatmeal
- ❖ Cut in wedges. Then coat with olive oil and seasonings for healthy baked sweet potato fries
- ❖ Mash sweet potatoes for a creamy alternative to white mashed potatoes (see recipe below)

NOTE: There are two types of sweet potato: moist (orange fleshed) and dry (yellow fleshed). The moist fleshed are often called Yams, but this is a misnomer as true Yams are a very large root vegetable grown in Africa and Asia and are rarely seen in the Western world.

Vanilla Cinnamon Mashed Sweet Potatoes:

Basic Preparation: Cook Sweet Potatoes + Add Liquid + Season + Blend + Bake

Ingredients:

3 large sweet potatoes (or yams if you prefer)

½ teaspoon cinnamon

½ teaspoon vanilla

Vanilla Liquid Stevia, Powdered Stevia or sweetener of choice (to taste)

Small amount of low-fat milk or dairy substitute such as Almond Milk, if desired for extra creamy consistency

1-2 tablespoons butter or butter alternative (optional)

(serves 4-6)

- ❖ Bake sweet potatoes, with skins, on a cookie sheet at 375 degrees for about an hour until done (Pierce with fork to test doneness after about 45 minutes.) Or if you prefer, steam cubed sweet potatoes, without skins, in steamer until they are tender. (approx. 15-25 minutes.)
- ❖ Let potatoes cool. Then cut baked sweet potatoes in half and scoop out the potato flesh and put in a large bowl. Discard the skins. (if steamed, cool and place in bowl.)
- ❖ Add in the rest of the ingredients and mash the potato mixture with a potato masher. When blended, add the mixture to an electric blender or food processor and blend until the mixture is a smooth consistency. (add in batches if needed)
- ❖ Spoon mixture into a casserole dish. Sprinkle top very lightly with some extra cinnamon.
- ❖ Cover and bake for ½ hour to 40 minutes.

If desired, toast some chopped pecans and sprinkle them on top of the potatoes along with the cinnamon before baking.

Roasting Sweet Potatoes

Roasting sweet potatoes could not be easier. I usually roast up a batch on a Sunday and use them in a variety of recipes such as Sweet Potato Home Fries, Arugula Salad with Sweet Potatoes, Walnuts & Goat Cheese, or Sweet Potato Salad. (using sweet potatoes instead of the traditional white potatoes and a vinaigrette instead of mayonnaise)

On a cold winter day, I put them in oatmeal or when I get a sweet craving, I just eat them plain. For these types of recipes I cut the sweet potatoes in cubes. (you can also cut sweet potatoes in wedges as an alternative to French Fries). Both preparations are below.

Basic Preparation: Cut Potatoes in Desired Shape & Size + Coat with Oil & Seasonings + Roast

"Cubed" Roasted Sweet Potatoes.

* **Prepare**: You can leave the skins on for added taste & nutrients or peel the potatoes, try it both ways and see which you prefer. If you are leaving the skins on, scrub the potatoes well with a vegetable brush, and then dry them with a paper towel before slicing them. If you are peeling them, you should wash them first.

* **Cut**: On a cutting board, cut off and discard the ends of the potatoes. Then slice into rounds. (How thick depends on how big you want your cubes) I usually keep them about ½ inch in thickness. Then slice the round lengthwise & across to make the "cubes".

* **Coat with Oil & Seasonings**: Next, place the cubes into a bowl and drizzle with olive oil. (approximately 1 tablespoon). Don't drown them in oil. They should look glossy, but they shouldn't be sitting in a pool of olive oil.

* Optionally, if you want to bring out the sweetness of the potatoes, you can also drizzle a very small amount of Balsamic Vinegar over the potatoes. Then season with a pinch of good quality sea salt and some pepper or with your favorite seasoning mix. (I usually use a seasoning blend that contains a variety of herbs & spices.)

* **Mix**: Combine all the ingredients and make sure all of the potato cubes are well coated. (It's a little messy, but the best way to make sure all the potatoes are coated is to mix the ingredients with your hands).

* **Roast**: Preheat the oven to 400°. (Some chefs roast at a little higher temperature, 425°. Try, both ways to see what works best for you.) Place the sweet potato cubes onto the baking sheet in a single layer. You can put a piece of parchment paper on the baking sheet, which makes cleanup easier. You can also use a pyrex dish, but the higher the side of the dish, the more the potatoes will "steam" instead of roasting. Also, don't overcrowd the potatoes, as that will also cause them to steam and become more mushy on the outside. Bake for 30-45 minutes, turning every 10 minutes with spatula so that potatoes brown, but do not burn. Serve warm.

"Traditional French Fry Cut".

* If your sweet potato is large, first cut it in half. Next cut a thin slice from both ends. This will eliminate little pointy ends on your fries. Next, take a half of the sweet potato and cut it into large slices about 3/4 inch thick. You'll then cut the larger slices into fries. Your fries should be 1/2 inch to 3/4 inch thick.

* For a bigger wedge cut, peel the potatoes or you can leave the skins on. Just make sure the potatoes are well scrubbed. Cut the potato in half lengthwise, and cut each half into 6 wedges.

* Follow the roasting directions for "cubed" roasted sweet potatoes, above.

SMOOTHIES

The key ingredients for a delicious and healthy smoothie are:

Liquid + Protein/Fiber + Fruits and/or Vegetables + Thickener + .Other Flavorings/Nutrients

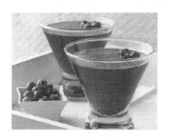

Then, you can add other extras for different tastes, health benefits, and textures. If you are using ice as a thickener, make sure you have a blender with enough power to crush the ice so that the ice doesn't remain in chunks and you get a nice smooth texture.

There is no right or wrong way to make a smoothie.

With one caveat, avoid ingredients high in sugar and/or fructose. if you want to fight cravings and are concerned about blood sugar control, stick with low glycemic fruits such as berries, and go easy on the bananas. Also, always try to add some protein or fiber.

Below are some options and ideas for combining ingredients to make a perfect smoothie.

LIQUID:
- ❖ Water
- ❖ Coconut Milk - Unsweetened
- ❖ Almond Milk-Unsweetened
- ❖ Other Nut Milk
- ❖ Rice Milk
- ❖ Fruit Juice-No sugar added (use sparingly)
- ❖ Vegetable Juice

FRUIT/VEGETABLES:
- ❖ Frozen Acai Berry Puree
- ❖ Blueberries
- ❖ Strawberries
- ❖ Raspberries
- ❖ Peaches
- ❖ Apple
- ❖ Slightly Ripe Banana
- ❖ Apples
- ❖ Carrots
- ❖ Kale
- ❖ Spinach
- ❖ Avocado

THICKENER:
- ❖ Ice
- ❖ Frozen Berries (Acai, Blueberries, or Strawberries)
- ❖ Frozen Banana (small portion, not overly ripe)
- ❖ Greek Yogurt (Plain/Unsweetened)
- ❖ Silken Tofu

OTHER:
- ❖ Greens Powder
- ❖ Acai Powder
- ❖ Goji Berry Powder
- ❖ Cacao Powder
- ❖ Cinnamon
- ❖ Vanilla
- ❖ Cacao Nibs
- ❖ Lecithin
- ❖ Dark Chocolate

PROTEIN/FIBER
- ❖ Protein Powder (such as Whey)
- ❖ Silken Tofu
- ❖ Yogurt (unsweetened)
- ❖ Ground Flax Seed
- ❖ Spirulina
- ❖ Brewer Yeast
- ❖ Chia Seeds (ground or whole)
- ❖ Almond Butter
- ❖ PGX Satisfast (Whey Protein Energy Drink with konjac-

SWEETENERS:
- ❖ Stevia (powder or liquid)
- ❖ Try different liquid stevia flavors….
- ❖ Truvia
- ❖ (Or other Sweetener of choice depending on your preferences & health)

Super Berry Smoothie:

Ingredients:

½ - 1 cup unsweetened Vanilla Almond Milk (depending on thickness*)

1-2 scoops of Vanilla Protein Powder (such as Whey Protein Powder)

2 teaspoons of almond butter

½ cup frozen blueberries (I like to use frozen wild blueberries)

1 packet frozen Acai Berry Puree

½ tsp cinnamon

1 1/2 tablespoons ground flax seed (optional)

4-6 Ice cubes (as desired, the more ice-cubes, the thicker the smoothie)

Directions:

❖ Pour the Almond Milk into a blender.

❖ Add the remaining ingredients

❖ Mix the ingredients in the blender until smooth.

❖ Pour into a glass and enjoy!

Choco-Green Smoothie:

Ingredients:

½ -1 cup low fat milk or unsweetened Chocolate Almond Milk

1-2 scoops of Chocolate Protein Powder (such as Whey Protein Powder)

2 teaspoons of almond butter

1 Scoop chocolate flavored Greens Powder

1 tbsp. raw Cacao powder

1 packet frozen Acai Berry Puree

1 tbsp. Goji Powder (optional)

4-6 Ice cubes (as desired, the more ice-cubes, the thicker the smoothie)

Sweetener (Try Powdered Stevia, fruit flavored Liquid Stevia or Truvia)

OPTIONAL:
Add a small amount of frozen blueberries for extra sweetness and antioxidants

Try adding a small amount of avocado for extra creaminess, additional fiber, and healthy monounsaturated fat.

Directions:

❖ Pour the milk into a blender.

❖ Add the remaining ingredients

❖ Mix the ingredients in the blender until smooth.

TIPS

❖ *If you like your smoothie thinner, use more Almond Milk

❖ *If you like a thicker smoothie, use less liquid and/or add ½ cup Greek yogurt

❖ If you like your smoothie to have a sweeter taste, add a small amount of sweetener of choice

❖ Want more antioxidants? Add some frozen Acai Berry Puree (Sambazon makes an organic, unsweetened puree)

Tips for Selecting Whey Protein Powder

Whey is a dairy protein that is a by-product of the cheese making process. In its raw state, whey contains substantial amounts of fat and lactose.

Whey Protein Powder is filtered and processed: to remove most of the lactose and fat.

There are two types of Whey protein products: Whey protein isolate and concentrate. The main difference is that the isolate is more pure. In other words, isolate contains more protein with less fat and lactose per serving.

When picking a Whey Protein Powder look for a product that:
•Is free of bovine growth hormones
•Has a good taste
•Mixes easily
•Contains no artificial chemical sweeteners
•Contains no refined carbohydrates such as fructose, sucrose or brown rice syrup

Introduction to the Glycemic Index

The Glycemic Index is a ranking of foods based on their immediate effect on blood sugar levels. Foods that break down quickly during digestion have the highest index values. The higher the GI of a food the faster the resultant rise in blood sugar after eating it, and the higher the GI, the higher the body's insulin response tends to be. Conversely, foods that break down slowly, releasing glucose gradually into the blood stream have a low index value. Selecting foods with lower GI levels promotes normal blood sugar levels, and enables the body to stay in a fat burning mode. For ease of use, you can think of foods as being in three general categories:

❖ High Index ratings -greater than 70

❖ Intermediate Index ratings-55 to 70 range

❖ Low Index ratings-below 55

The Glycemic Index is another tool for you to use when selecting foods to consume, but it is not an absolute. A variety of factors affect the glycemic response of individual foods, including, ❶ the type of carbohydrate (simple vs. complex), ❷ the degree to which the food is processed, and ❸ how the food is prepared.

Additionally the overall effect of a food on blood sugar levels will depend on the amount consumed and the foods consumed with it. A factor called the Glycemic Load, takes these additional elements into account.

Not all foods have been tested for their GI value. The GI listing of foods on the following pages is meant as a guideline. Knowing the exact GI or GL level of foods is not necessary in order to utilize the GI principles to guide your food choices. Having a general understanding of GI principles will help you when ratings are not available. Below are some general guidelines to follow when maintaining a low GI food plan. For a list of websites where you can find more detailed GI food listings and additional information about the Glycemic Index, visit the Resource page at www.diabetescoaching.com.

Using the Glycemic Index to your advantage:

Eat lots of non-starchy vegetables and low index legumes. Vegetables are a cornerstone of good health. Legumes/beans are nutritious and generally rich in soluble fibers which form a thick gel when mixed with water. This slows their passage through the digestive tract and contributes to the low GI of these foods.

Go easy on starchy vegetables which tend to be higher on the GI Index. These include white potato, (mashed, baked boiled, fried), parsnips, & corn.

Avoid grain-based flour products and consider the level of processing and type of starch. The less processed and rougher the grain, the lower the GI will be. Additionally, there are two types of starch in foods, amylase and amylopectin. Foods with more amylose tend to have a lower glycemic index. certain types of rice including American long grain rice and Basmati rice are lower on the index because of their higher amylose content. (you should still eat rice sparingly)

Add something acidic. The naturally occurring acids in certain fruits, as well as the acids in fermented foods like yogurt, buttermilk and sourdough breads slow the rate of digestion and contribute to the low GI of these foods. Additionally, adding vinegar or lemon juice to a food can help slow their conversion to glucose in the bloodstream.

Avoid lowering the GI of food by adding saturated fat to your diet. Although the presence of fat lowers the GI of a food or meal by slowing the rate at which it leaves the stomach, adding saturated fats to your food is not the best way to lower the GI Index of a food. (Adding a small amount of "good for you" fat such as olive oil is a good choice, on occasion.)

Consider the glycemic load and all of the nutritional qualities of a food before rejecting or consuming it. For example carrots and pumpkin are higher on the GI index, but have a low glycemic load and significant nutritional value. If you have blood sugar issues, the key is to eat carrots and pumpkin in moderation. Likewise, Peanut M&M's are low on the glycemic index, but are generally not a good choice for maintaining optimal health

Glycemic Index Guide
Vegetables and Salad Greens

Low GI	Medium GI	High GI
ENJOY- "Eat a Rainbow"	**Eat Occasionally**	**Avoid**
Alfalfa sprouts		
Artichokes	Beets	Baked Potato
Asparagus	Corn	French Fries
Avocado (1/4 slice)	Red Bliss Potato (mashed, baked, boiled)	Hashed Browns (made with white potatoes)
Bean Sprouts	Yam or sweet potato	Potato Chips (medium-high, avoid)
Bell peppers (red, green, yellow)	Winter Squash (acorn, butternut, spaghetti)	Parsnips(med-high-avoid)
Bok Choy		
Broccoli	Tomato Juice (1/2 cup); Tomato Paste (2 TBSP) Tomato Sauce (1/2 cup, no sugar added)	
Brussels sprouts		
Cabbage (red or white); Sauerkraut (no sugar added		
Cauliflower	*Pumpkin: (has a high glycemic index but relatively low glycemic load)	
Celery		
Cucumber		
Eggplant		
Green Beans		
Hot peppers		
Jicama		
Leafy Greens (Arugula, Collard Greens, Dandelion Greens, Endive, Kale, Parsley, Spinach, Watercress)		
Lettuce, all types		
Leeks		
Mushrooms		
Okra		
Olives (limit to 5)		
Onions		
Radishes		
Snow Peas		
Water Chestnuts		
Yellow Squash		
Zucchini		

Grains, Cereals & Baked Goods

Low GI	Medium GI	High GI
* eat sparingly & with vegetables and/or protein	* eat sparingly & with vegetables and/or protein	AVOID:
Quinoa	Sprouted Grain Bread (3+ grams of fiber)	White Rice/Arborio Rice
Pearled Barley	All Bran/Fiber One	All white flour products (including pasta)
Buckwheat (Kasha-Groats)	Brown Rice	Grain-based flour products including:
	Basmati Rice	Bagels
	Couscous	Cookies
	Grape Nuts	Cereal
	Muesli or Granola (no sugar added)	
	Steel Cut/Old Fashioned Oatmeal	
	Whole Grain Pasta	

Fruit

Low GI	Medium GI	High GI
Best Choice:	**Avoid**	**Avoid**
¾ cup berries (blueberries/strawberries, raspberries, blackberries, boysenberries)	Apricots, 4 medium	Cantaloupe 1/3, small)
Lemon	Dates (fresh), 2	Grapes, ½ cup
Small Portions/occasionally	Figs (fresh), 2	Honeydew melon (1/4 of a medium melon)
Apple	½ Pineapple (raw)	Raisins (2 tbsp.)
4 medium apricots	Less ripe banana	Watermelon (¾ cup)
12 large cherries		Very ripe banana
Grapefruit		Canned fruits in syrup
Guava		
Kiwi		
Kumquats, 4 medium		
Mandarin orange		
Regular orange (small)		
½ small mango		
Nectarine		
½ medium papaya		
Peach		
Pear		
½ of a small pomegranate		

Protein

Best Choices for Low GI Eating	Eat in Moderation or Sparingly:	Avoid
Canned salmon, or sardines packed in water Chicken, turkey, or hen (skinless) Fresh fish Seafood (shrimp, scallops, clams, lobster, calamari, squid, octopus, mussels etc.) Tofu, tempeh Veggie or Garden Burger (low fat) Nuts (walnuts, pecans, almonds, Brazil Nuts) Lentils Beans (red, black, garbanzo, lima, adzuki, pinto, soy) Omega 3 Eggs Protein Powder (no sugar added)	Cashews (low/medium- eat sparingly) Canadian Bacon Lean red meat (beef, pork, lamb, etc.)	Salami, Bacon/nitrates, Hot Dogs, Beef Pastrami High Fat Red Meat

Dairy & Substitutes

Best Choices for Low GI Eating	Eat in Moderation or Sparingly:	Avoid
Oat or nut milk (Low-fat/Non-fat, no sugar added) Plain Yogurt (Greek) Soy Yogurt (plain or flavored, Low-fat, no sugar added) Low Fat Cheese	Light Cream Cheese Light Sour Cream Skim or 1% Milk Part Skim Ricotta	Whole fat cheese Regular Cottage Cheese Cream Cheese Regular Sour Cream Whole fat yogurt Whole Milk Cream Whipped Cream

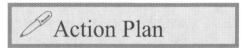

Putting Your Food Plan into Action

❖ **Get support.** You have many options, including working with a health counselor, diabetes coach, dietician, trainer, joining a support group or just teaming up with a friend. (A word of caution: be wary of fad diets or programs that don't meet your long term objectives.)

❖ **Take the Veggie Challenge.** Do you know how many servings of vegetables you eat in a day? A week? Use a daily journal and note how many vegetables you consume in a day or seven day time period. The results might surprise you.

❖ **Start keeping a daily food journal.** Keeping a food journal will help you to get a handle on what you are "really" eating throughout the day and allow you to observe both your food choices and patterns of eating that affect your blood sugars.

❖ **Each week select a vegetable that you don't eat regularly and add it to one of your meals.** Good choices include: Asparagus, broccoli, Brussels sprouts, cabbage, cauliflower, celery, collard greens, cucumber, kale, onions, green and red peppers, tomatoes, zucchini, and carrots, (note: although carrots are higher on the glycemic index, they are a good source of nutrients and OK in moderation).

❖ **Limit your intake of "starchy" vegetables, particularly white potatoes.** Sweet potatoes, yams, peas, turnips – also starchy vegetables - are lower on the glycemic index than white potatoes and are good sources of nutrients.

❖ **Become familiar with the different types of sweeteners.** Experiment with different sweeteners so that you can identify those that don't adversely affect your blood sugars and determine which ones lead you towards your vision of health.

❖ **Each week select one of the Tips for Cutting Back on Sugar.** Do this on a regular basis until you are comfortable with the amount of sweeteners in your diet.

❖ **Eliminate Grain-based flour products.** The next time you have a sandwich, try Sprouted Grain or a bread made with nut, bean, golden flaxseed or coconut flour. (or a combination of any of these flours. Sometime referred to as "Paleo Bread".

❖ **Try substitutions for rice.** The next time you plan to eat rice, try quinoa or "cauliflower rice".

❖ **Try something different for breakfast.** There are no set rules for what to eat for breakfast. The key is to start the day with a breakfast that does not cause a sharp rise in blood sugars and that will satisfy you, setting the stage for healthy eating throughout the rest of the day.

❖ **Stock your work environment with healthy snacks.** The work environment is stressful, and that 4 p.m. "gotta have a snack" craving will get you every time if you are not prepared. Nut and seed mixes, low-fat cheese, almond butter with a slice of Paleo bread, or vegetables with dip are all good alternatives to the vending machine.

❸ Validate Your New Health Strategy with an Action Plan

Knowing what to do, and how to do it, are both critical components of conquering diabetes. But without action, knowledge will not take you very far. That is why you need to:

❖ Develop and commit to an action plan with goals and activities that support those goals

❖ Use your action plan to your advantage during those times when the going gets tough to help you get back on track.

Why Your Action Plan is the Key to Success

Your action plan will give you direction and keep you moving towards your goals. One of the things you will learn on the following pages is that there is a world of difference between committing to a plan that is written and trying to stick with a set of desires that you keep in your head.

Life is messy. The best thought out plans can go awry. If you don't exercise for a couple of days or the bag of Doritos and some French fries get the best of you, don't panic or berate yourself.

What do you need to do when you find yourself off-track? Use your written action plan to GET BACK TO BASICS.

When you find life getting in your way, setting goals and using a daily journal to reinforce success habits will be tools that you can rely on to reinforce positive lifestyle choices.

It is not necessary to work your plan perfectly. Think of your success habits as miles traveled on a winding road that will lead you to your destination of health. At times, you may find yourself on the side of the road. But, as long as you keep the road you have chosen in sight, you will be able to get back to it at your own pace, and you will ultimately reach the goals that you have set out for yourself.

On the following pages, you will learn how to develop an action plan that will ensure your success.

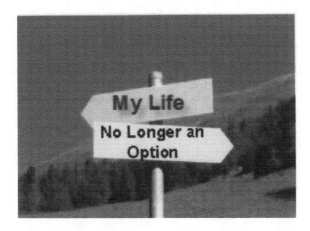

The Goal Setting Process

The goal setting process involves charting a plan for long term recovery as well as managing your day-to-day diabetes or pre-diabetes care. Setting goals and then accomplishing them with an action plan is crucial for improving your health and accomplishing what you want in your personal life. There is a direct relationship between goals and achievements because:

❖ Well-defined goals provide direction and help you achieve your desired results,

❖ Written goals provide you with a means of measuring progress, and

❖ Setting priorities keeps you focused and moving ahead on a steady path.

The goal setting process should ultimately:

❖ Identify long and short term goals which are broken down into manageable sub-parts so that progress can be measured,

❖ Provide a framework that will assist you in identifying priorities and activities to help you reach your goals,

❖ Set forth reasonably attainable goals as well as goals that are a stretch, so that you will experience ongoing positive feedback and a sense of accomplishment, and

❖ Provide you with a source of information that can be used to monitor and adjust ongoing behaviors.

Reviewing goals on a regular basis makes it easier for you to fine tune your efforts and helps you identify non-productive activities that can be abandoned. The information and exercises on the following pages will show you what is involved in the goal setting process and how to develop a set of goals that support your vision of health.

The Steps In The Goal Setting Process Are A Follows:

❖ Developing your unique vision which serves as the foundation for your action plan.

❖ Sketch out a plan for achieving your desired results.

❖ Translate your plan into concrete goals and sub-goals that support your vision.

❖ Define activities to help you take consistent actions towards your goals.

❖ Identify any obstacles and develop strategies for overcoming these roadblocks.

❖ Follow through with a commitment contract.

Developing your Vision

What your mind can conceive of and believe, it can achieve. Vision is the key to self-motivation. In his book Unlimited Power, Anthony Robbins reminds us that "People who succeed know what they want and believe they can get it."

In order to develop an effective plan for conquering diabetes or pre-diabetes, it is absolutely essential that you develop clarity about where you are and where you want to go. In order to develop a vision that will propel you towards your goals, you must:

✓ See It	✓ Own It	✓ Want It	✓ Believe It

Your Vision

Conquering diabetes or pre-diabetes is not just about what you eat. Your vision will also include other hopes and aspirations relating to your career, physical activity and relationships. Joshua Rosenthal, founder of the Institute of Integrative Nutrition, refers to these as "primary foods". These are your dreams, they are what feed your spirituality and if you believe in them, they will come true.

One way to think about your life vision is to identify qualities you would like to develop, things you would like to do, and things you would like to have as a healthy person with your blood sugars under control. Part of your vision will be directly related to your physical health, while other aspects will include things you hope to achieve as part of your overall life plan. Below are some examples:

Qualities I Would Like to DEVELOP:
- ❖ I would like to be more energetic
- ❖ I would like to be focused
- ❖ I would like to be physically fit

Things I Would Like to DO:
- ❖ I would like to lose weight
- ❖ I would like to go back to school to learn how to be a chef
- ❖ I would like to take a year off of work and travel

Things I Would Like to HAVE:
- ❖ I would like to have my own business
- ❖ I would like to have a garden to grow my own vegetables
- ❖ I would like to have more friends and time to spend with them

The exercises on the following pages are designed to help you identify your vision and to determine if you are ready to move forward with recommended lifestyle changes. If you find yourself resistant, they will help you to examine what is standing in your way.

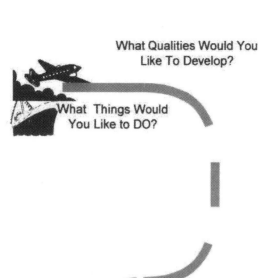

What Qualities Would You
Like To Develop?

What Things Would
You Like to DO?

Your Vision is your roadmap for
where you want to go in your life.

Thinking about the questions on this
page will help you to gain clarity
about where you are and how you
see your life unfolding in the future.

What Things
Would You Like
to Have?

Where Do You Want to Live?

What relationships
would you like to have in
your life?

What Are Your Top 3
Health Goals?

What Would You
Like Your Life's
Work To Be?

Activities for Strengthening Your Vision, Developing Mental Clarity, and Exploring Your Spirituality

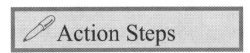 Action Steps

Set Forth a Vision of Your Life as a "Healthy" Person

❖ Remember, good health is a state of complete physical, mental, social and spiritual well-being, and not merely an absence of disease. Start brainstorming How much would you like to weigh, what type of food plan would you like to incorporate into your lifestyle, what would you like to be doing 1 year, 5 years, 10 years from now?

❖ From this vision you will be able to set concrete goals and communicate your vision to your medical care providers so that they can assist you to reach your vision of health. If you are having trouble coming up with your vision statement, try the exercise on the preceding page as a starting point.

Write In Your Journal.

❖ An effective technique when you are feeling stuck is to spend 5-10 minutes in the morning writing whatever comes to mind. There is no right or wrong way to write these thoughts in your journal. The point is to let your conscious mind go and let yourself express emotions and feelings that are holding you back. If you write faithfully in your journal first thing in the morning for a period of time, you will find a greater connection to the source of wisdom within you that will help you claim the life you want to lead.

Create a Vision Board

❖ A vision board is a visual representation or collage of the things you want to have, be or do in your life. Typically it consists of a poster or foam board with cut-out pictures, drawings and/or writing on it of the things that represent your desires, objectives, dreams and goals. There are also companies that provide software programs so that you can create an electronic vision board. The purpose of creating a vision board is to start the process of attracting the events and circumstances into your life that will enable you to manifest your vision so that it becomes a reality.

❖ Your vision board can be very simple or complex. The key elements of a vision board are 1) a visual design that stimulates your mind 2) pictures and words that evoke a positive emotional response 3) location in a strategic place for maximum exposure

Seek Assistance.

❖ If journaling or other techniques are not sufficient, and you feel depressed or unable to make needed changes to improve your health, seek assistance from your primary physician or enlist assistance from other sources such as a counselor or diabetes coach.

In some cases, very powerful beliefs about ourselves developed over a lifetime can inhibit our ability to live the life we desire. The book "The Power of Belief" by Ray Dodd explores these issues and provides a roadmap for identifying beliefs holding you back and for putting new beliefs in their place. This can be a good place to start if you feel stuck, and it can be helpful to work through this process with a life coach.

How to Translate Goals into an Action Plan

❖ **Identify your goals and put them in writing**. Thinking about your goals is very different from writing them down. Articulating goals and putting them in writing provides clarity and demonstrates a commitment to achieving your goals. Goals that stay in your head usually become confusing and are easily abandoned. Written goals tend to be more specific than unwritten goals and are more likely to be achieved.

❖ **Divide your goals into sub-goals**. These are steps or achievements you will strive to accomplish on the way to achieving the main goal. Then, identify activities that will promote the achievement of each sub-goal. Sub-goals provide an objective method of measuring your progress toward the main goal and show you where you may have to make adjustments. Achieving sub-goals also provides you with a sense of confidence that will encourage you to keep moving forward toward attainment of your ultimate goal.

❖ **Define activities to help you take consistent actions towards your goals.** The activities that promote the achievement of each sub-goal become the building blocks that are the foundation for your goals and the criteria for measuring your progress.

❖ **Identify any obstacles that you perceive as getting in your way of achieving your goals and ultimately your life vision.** To overcome obstacles, ask yourself empowering questions that will lead you towards solutions that will help you to move forward. If you have deep seated beliefs that are holding you back, now is the time to uncover the roots of those beliefs. Explore techniques such as those in Ray Dodd's book "The Power of Belief" to put aside limiting beliefs that no longer serve you.

❖ **Establish reasonable deadlines for achieving your goals**. Setting deadlines provides closure and ensures that a particular goal does not remain unattended for too long a time period. Too many open-ended activities can be frustrating, leaving one with a sense of not getting anything done.

❖ **Learn to distinguish goals from open-ended desires**. If you have trouble committing a goal to writing, it probably isn't a goal but an open-ended desire (that you may or may not be able to translate into a goal). Sometimes, as you attempt to list the activities that will help you achieve a particular goal, you may find that you simply do not want to engage in those activities. When this happens, you may decide to postpone that goal or abandon it altogether.

❖ **Review your goals regularly, and be willing to revise your goals and abandon unreasonable goals.** Just setting a goal does not guarantee that you will achieve it. But, if you have followed all of the steps listed above, it will guarantee that you will be moving steadily forward, toward the articulated goal. Sometimes as you work through your sub-goals, you will determine that the end goal no longer makes sense. Perhaps an event has occurred that no longer makes the goal a priority. Remember that goals represent the way you see your life from today's perspective. Monitor your progress as you go, and change your goals as your perspective changes.

The Anatomy of A Goal

The goal is written, measurable and has a deadline.

__Goal__: Lose 30 lbs. in 6 months

The goal is broken down into reasonable sub-goals.

__Sub-Goal__: Lose 10% of body weight in 2 months

Activities are identified that will lead you towards the goal.

These activities can be specified in more detail as success habits to practice on a daily basis. In order to identify activities, you can ask yourself empowering questions associated with your goals or sub-goals. Example: What do I need to do in order lose 10% of my body weight in 2 months?

If you see an obstacle to meeting a goal or completing an activity, ask yourself what you can do to overcome that obstacle and write those activities down as well.

❖ Walk 30 minutes at brisk pace 6 days per week

❖ Go to gym and use weights 2 days per week

❖ Develop food plan and follow it daily

❖ Cut out refined carbohydrates

What is one health related goal you would like to attain? Is this goal a MUST?

Goal:

Sub-Goals:

Activities:

❖

❖

❖

❖

Are there any obstacles to obtaining your goals or completing activities? What do you need to do to overcome those obstacles?

Use this page to list any other goals you would like to reach as you improve your health.

Goal:

Sub-Goals:

Activities:

* ❖
* ❖
* ❖
* ❖
* ❖
* ❖
* ❖

Goal:

Sub-Goals:

Activities:

* ❖
* ❖
* ❖
* ❖
* ❖

❹ Establish New Success Habits

Controlling diabetes is challenging because there is no quick fix. It requires making changes that will enable you to keep your blood sugar under control and complications at bay for the rest of your life.

> **Motivation is what gets you started.**
> **Habit is what keeps you going**
> *Jim Ryun*

It is not necessary to make drastic changes. In fact, there are lots of *"little"* things you can do that can make a *"big"* difference in your overall health. The trick is to develop a daily routine that takes into account the nutrients that you put into your body, your level of activity, and a way to monitor your progress.

The first part of this chapter will provide you with insights to help you understand how to change habits that are holding you back from reaching your health goals and how to put new habits in their place.

You have already learned how to put a Food Plan in place to support your body with nutritious foods that support blood sugar control. In the second part of this chapter, we are going to help you to implement new daily habits that will support your food plan in the areas of exercise and stress management. These new success habits are summarized below.

EXERCISE & MANAGING STRESS

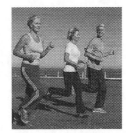

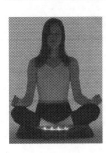

* ❖ Exercise regularly. (Just 20-30 minutes a day of aerobic exercise can be very beneficial) Add strength training to build muscle. Try to build up to 1 Hour of exercise at least 3-5 days a week.

* ❖ Manage stress in your daily life. (For example, with deep breathing, meditation, or Yoga)

* ❖ Practice Gratitude. (Studies are beginning to show that experiencing gratitude in our daily lives has a positive impact both on stress levels and overall health.)

Success Habits Part I: How to Change a Habit

❖ Habits are the fabric of your life.

❖ Your daily behaviors take you either towards or away from your vision of health

❖ Success habits support your well-being and lead you towards your goals

❖ People who achieve their goals avoid or minimize activities and behaviors that lead them away from their vision and maximize behaviors that lead them forward.

In their essence, success habits are repeated behaviors that eventually become automatic. Many of us have the idea that we need to do something extraordinary to make meaningful changes in our lives. Paradoxically, it's the little things that you do on a daily basis that determine your success.

In this chapter, you will learn new behaviors that will help you to successfully manage your blood sugars. But knowing what to do is just one half of the equation. Understanding how to make changes, particularly when old habits are getting in your way is the key to success.

In order to change or eliminate a habit that is holding you back you need to be:	Steps for changing a habit include:
❖ Aware of the habit and its effect. ❖ Self-motivated to change the habit, and ❖ Willing to take action to change the habit.	❖ Identifying the habits holding you back from attaining your vision, ❖ Identifying new habits to put in their place, and ❖ Taking action by practicing new habits.

The first step in changing behavior is self-awareness. To enable my clients to gain greater clarity about their everyday habits, I created an assessment exercise that is designed to uncover key behaviors that affect blood sugar management. As individuals move through the coaching program, they can refer back to this exercise in order to identify habits holding them back and then make effective changes.

Have fun with this exercise. Do not "over think" your responses. There are no right or wrong answers. Remember, you can't change a habit until you are fully conscious of the behavior. With that in mind, the main purpose of the exercise is to bring your habits to your full awareness and to get you thinking about what you eat, how you exercise and how you manage your health on a day to day basis.

My clients like to take the assessment at the beginning of their coaching program and then again at the end. The diagram provides them with a visual of how much their habits have changed, and they are amazed at their progress over the course of the program.

Instructions for how to complete the exercise are set forth on the following page.

Success Habits Assessment

Answer each question in the Success Habits Assessment. Then, based on your answer, either circle the color that corresponds to your response in the Circle of Success Habits™ diagram or use a crayon, marker or colored pencil to fill in the appropriate color.

Example: How often do you eat the following categories of foods:		
Vegetables	4-9 servings of non-starchy vegetables (do not include white potatoes, corn, turnips)	● Rarely/Occasionally (Red) ○ 3-5 days per week (Yellow) ● Everyday (Green)

If you generally eat 4-9 servings of non-starchy vegetables 3-5 days per week, then in the Vegetable section, either circle the letter "Y" or color in the space using a yellow marker or crayon.

As you fill in your responses, a visual pattern begins to emerge that will show you:

❖ Habits where you are on track, (GREEN)

❖ Habits where you might want to make adjustments, (YELLOW) and

❖ Habits that are likely holding you back from meeting your objectives. (RED

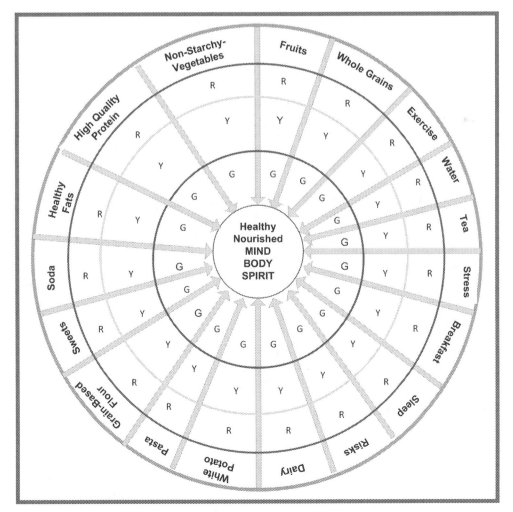

123

Success Habits Assessment

Foods To Eat More Of:		
How often do you eat the following categories of foods?		
Vegetables	4-9 servings of non-starchy vegetables. (do not include white potatoes, corn, turnips) (50% of daily food intake)	● Rarely Occasionally (Red)
High Quality Protein	One or more of the following: Protein powder, tofu, organic/Free Range chicken or turkey, eggs or egg whites (organic), Wild salmon, tilapia, sardines, flounder, catfish, tuna etc. (do not include shell fish), Beans, Yogurt, Kefir	◐ 3-5 days per week (Yellow)
Healthy Fats	Combination of Nuts, ¼ cup (do not include cashews or peanuts) Seeds, (Ground Flax, Chia, Pumpkin, Sunflower, Sesame) Other Healthy Fats, (Avocado, Cold Pressed Olive Oil)	● Everyday (Green)
FOODS TO EAT Sparingly: How often do you eat the following categories of foods?		
Whole Grains	Rice, Barley, Oats, Quinoa, Millet, Rye etc..	● Everyday (Red)
High Fat Dairy/Red Meat	Butter, Cream, Whole Milk, Cheese (other than low fat), Whole Milk, Regular Sour Cream, Regular Cottage Cheese, High Fat non-grass fed Red Meat	◐ 3-5 days per week, (Yellow)
Fruit	Medium Glycemic Fruit (see list on page 93) High Glycemic Fruit (very ripe bananas, raisins, cantaloupe, honeydew melon, watermelon, grapes ½ cup, canned in syrup)	◑ Occasionally (G)
FOODS TO AVOID: How often do you eat the following categories of foods?		
White Potato	Baked Potato, Mashed Potatoes, French Fries	● Everyday (Red)
Pasta	Any type of pasta made with grain-based flour	◐ 3-5 days per week, (Yellow)
Grain-Based Flour	Includes any product that has grain-based flour such as bread, crackers, cake, cookies	◑ Occasionally (G)
Sweets	Includes consumption of sugar or artificial sweeteners.	
Soda	Includes both regular and "diet" soda	
BEHAVIORS: How Often Do You Engage in the Following Activities?		
Exercise	½ HR to 1 Hour of Exercise (Aerobic, Strength Training)	● Rarely Occasionally (Red)
Water	Consume 6-8 servings of water	
Tea	Drink tea (green or black)	◐ 3-5 days per week (Yellow)
Stress Management	½ HR to 1 Hour (Yoga, Stretching, Meditation, Personal Time, Deep Breathing etc.)	● Everyday (Green)
Breakfast	Consisting of one or more of the following; non-starchy vegetables; healthy protein, low glycemic fruit, low-fat dairy or dairy substitute; occasional cooked quinoa or oats, low glycemic fruit smoothie/green smoothie/green drink	
Sleep	7-8 Hours Restful Sleep	

Circle of Success Habits™

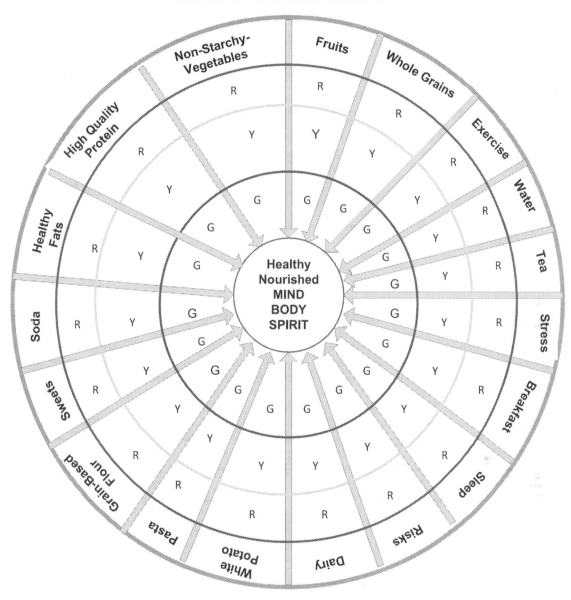

Risk Factors For Diabetes

- ❖ Family History
- ❖ 20% over a healthy weight or obese
- ❖ Sedentary Lifestyle
- ❖ You are African-American, Latino, Asian, Native American or Pacific Islander
- ❖ Diabetes during pregnancy or giving birth to a baby weighing 9 pounds (or more)
- ❖ Low HDL (good cholesterol) or high overall cholesterol levels
- ❖ Very high blood pressure or very high triglycerides

⬤ 3+ Risk Factors (Red)

◖ 2-3 Risk Factors (Yellow)

⬤ 0-1 Risk Factors (Green)Low HDL (good cholesterol) or high overall cholesterol levels

© 2014, Great Life, Inc

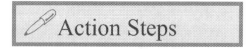 Action Steps

Identifying Habits that Are Holding You Back

❖ Are you able to see any patterns emerging that shed light on behaviors that are holding you back from achieving your health goals?

❖ What habits can you identify that are holding you back?

❖ Select one habit you would like to change. Write the habit you are willing to change in your journal and develop a game plan for putting a new habit in its place.

❖ If you repeat this process, over the course of six months to a year, you will have made significant lifestyle changes - one success habit at a time.

❖ If you have identified a habit that you are finding particularly hard to change, try using the STOP method on the following pages to help you to understand the link between your thoughts, feelings and subsequent behaviors. This will help you to break through the issues holding you back from making changes that you desire.

❖ Take An Attitude Check. When you find yourself saying "I can't" to a suggestion or an idea that could improve your condition, substitute the words "I don't want to" or "I am not ready to" adopt that behavior. Notice the shift that occurs when you take responsibility for your actions and the space it creates to find a solution.

To help you brainstorm, below are examples of common habits that might be holding you back and success habits that will lead you towards your vision of health. Are any of these habits that you would like to change?

Old Habit	New Success Habit
FOOD HABITS	
❖ Drink cup of coffee in the morning	❖ Drink cup of green tea first thing in the morning
❖ Skip breakfast	❖ Plan ahead and make time to eat breakfast
❖ Eat white bread	❖ Eat whole grain bread
❖ Eat after 8 pm in evening	❖ Have cup of tea in evening and skip late night snack
❖ Drink soda with meals	❖ Drink water or green tea with meals
❖ Eat when you are anxious, bored, angry, etc.	❖ Substitute another activity for eating when you are anxious, bored, angry, etc.
EXERCISE HABITS	
❖ Stay up late at night so that you are too tired to get up early to do exercise	❖ Go to bed earlier so that you can wake up in morning and fit in exercise
❖ Overbook schedule leaving no time for exercise	❖ Plan weekly and schedule in daily exercise at a time that works for you
❖ Sit and watch TV	❖ Walk on treadmill, peddle on exercise bike, or jump on re-bounder while watching TV
❖ Always take the elevator	❖ When possible take the stairs
❖ Skip exercise when it is raining or snowing	❖ Buy videos and exercise indoors

The Power of Exercise

Any level of exercise reduces your risk of getting diabetes, and if you are already diagnosed, exercise is one of the most powerful ways to make your body more receptive to insulin. Getting moving should be an integral part of every diabetic's recovery plan, keeping in mind your current level of physical activity and any limitations that should be discussed with your doctor before starting an exercise program. Incorporating exercise into your daily routine will provide a number of benefits, including clearing the blood of glucose, increasing insulin sensitivity, and improving heart and cardiovascular health.

Activity lowers blood glucose levels in two ways:

❖ First, it causes your cells to become more sensitive to insulin. What this means is that your insulin is more effective, and hence more glucose is used by your cells. This sensitivity to insulin and the benefit of lower blood glucose levels lasts for several hours, even after the activity has ended.

❖ Second, it lowers the amount of glucose produced in the liver. In addition to getting glucose from the food you eat, you also get glucose from the liver. This is a normal function of the liver, but sometimes it makes more glucose than your body can use, causing your blood glucose level to go up. Regular activity can help counter this effect.

When thinking about what types of activities to include, you can break exercise into a number of categories:

❖ *Physical Activity,* which is any movement that uses energy such as climbing the stairs, mowing the lawn or walking an extra row in the parking lot to get to your car.

❖ *Aerobic Exercise* that can be thought of as more vigorous, continuous and concerted movement like dancing, walking, running, rebounding or bicycling.

❖ *Recreational Activities* such as golf, bowling, tennis, hiking.

❖ *Flexibility and Strength Activities* which are very beneficial for relieving emotional tension and stress. Examples of these activities include stretching, yoga, tai chi, and strength training with weights.

Ideally, your overall plan should include all four exercise categories over the course of a week. But, if you are not already active, just getting started with some extra physical activity will be beneficial. Exactly how often you should and can exercise depends on many factors including your:

❖ Overall health,

❖ Blood glucose levels and control,

❖ Lifestyle, and

❖ Diabetes complications, if relevant.

Once you have approval from your doctor, at least thirty to sixty minutes of continuous exercise every day will pay off in enhanced health. The important thing is to make exercise part of your daily routine in a way that supports your lifestyle and vision of health.

Exercise Safety Guidelines for Diabetics

❖ Rule #1: Clear any exercise program with your physician. This is absolutely essential for diabetics. In addition to assessing your overall physical health, your doctor can determine the kinds of exercise that are right for you. This decision will take into account certain kinds of exercise you should avoid if you have diabetic complications such as retinopathy, heart disease, or nerve damage.

❖ Start any new exercise routine slowly, with a gradual build up. For example, if you are starting a walking program, begin with just 10 minutes a day and gradually work up to 30 or 60 minutes a day.

❖ Stop whenever you don't feel well. If you feel pain or pressure in any area of your body during the exercise activity or experience shakiness, dizziness, faintness, blurry vision or headaches, discontinue the activity and inform your physician.

❖ Be consistent. You will get better results and you will avoid injury if you make some form of exercise part of your daily routine.

❖ Drink plenty of fluids. This is important for anyone participating in an exercise session, whether or not you have diabetes. Drink before exercise, during exercise if it's longer than 20 minutes, and afterward.

❖ Make attentive foot care an integral part of your exercise program. Peripheral nerve damage can lead to a loss of sensation in the feet, which means that a blister can go unnoticed and become infected. To avoid problems with your feet, buy fitness shoes that fit well, break them in slowly, and wear clean socks every time you exercise. After exercising, make sure to check your feet for blisters, redness or tenderness, and talk with your health care team if you experience any of these problems.

❖ Learn how your body responds to particular types of exercise by checking your blood glucose levels before, during, and after exercise.

❖ Know the symptoms of hypoglycemia. When exercising, keep a quick source of carbohydrates or other food that is recommended by your health care provider with you in the event that you suffer a quick or unexpected drop in blood sugar.

📖 *Reflections*

Janet: I exercise at least 30-60 minutes every day, incorporating activities that fit my lifestyle into my routine. Working 40-50 hours a week, at first I found it difficult to fit exercise into my schedule. What I find works best for me is to wake up ½ hour earlier to start my day with some stretching and yoga. I like to do my walking after work, but initially found that once I arrived home, I was distracted or too tired to exercise. But, I discovered that if I brought my exercise clothes with me to work and changed into them before leaving work, I was ready to go and mentally ready to get moving once I got home. Or sometimes, I will just walk for an hour downtown and then head home. For the first year after my diagnosis, I found exercise made a big difference in my energy and my glucose levels and it continues to be a mainstay of my diabetes management plan.

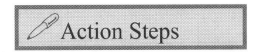

Action Steps

Getting Started With an Exercise Routine

* **Find Out How Active You Really Are:** A great way to find out where you stand is to invest in a pedometer. If you are taking less than 10,000 steps a day, set goals for getting more steps into your day. (Average your step counts for 3 days. Then determine how many steps you would need to average 10,000 steps per day.) If you are already close to or at 10,000 steps per day and want to become more active, develop a plan for adding 7,500 steps to your baseline. There are studies showing that people who use a pedometer to build more activity into their routine are more motivated to become more active in general and begin to see improvements in weight, cholesterol levels, body fat and overall fitness.

* **Identify Some Exercise Activities You Would Like to Try**: Think about what would fit into your daily routine. Some people enjoy getting out and going to the gym. Others would much prefer to take a walk in the park. Write down some activities that you think you "would actually do" and visualize when and how often you would do that activity in a week. Set goals that work for you. Plan to begin gradually and increase the intensity and duration of your workouts over time.

* **Make A Schedule:** It's easy to allow busy schedules and other activities to interfere with an activity plan. To avoid breaking your momentum, develop an exercise schedule and make it a priority. Consider carefully what times of the day and which days of the week are best for your activity. Think of your exercise time as a date you make with yourself, one that you wouldn't break or ignore anymore than you would consciously miss an appointment with someone else. If you find it helpful, write your activity schedule down in a calendar or daily planner.

* **Be Flexible**: Having said how important it is to make a schedule, it is also important not to make yourself crazy over exercising. If you do, you may grow to resent it and find yourself avoiding it altogether. The important thing is to keep moving on a regular basis. If you miss a day or two, the best thing you can do is to engage in some form of activity to get back into your routine, and don't beat yourself up for taking a few days off from exercising.

* **Find a Buddy:** Activities and exercise are often more fun when you do them with someone else. Also, a partner can help you stay motivated and give you someone to compare your progress with.

* **Build in Variety**: The worst thing that you can do is become so bored with your exercise routine that you don't want to do it. The best way to avoid this is to find several different types of activities that you enjoy and do them on different days of the week. You can even make your time in front of the TV count by working out on an exercise bike or treadmill while you watch your favorite show.

* **Try Rebounding**: Rebounding applies weight and movement to every cell, causing the entire body to become stronger and more flexible. It's fun, and rebounding is great for diabetics because it increases circulation, strengthens the heart, muscles and bones, and improves cell efficiency. Check with your doctor to make sure it is a form of exercise that is OK for you, and make sure you invest in a high quality rebound unit that is designed properly so that you won't sustain injuries to your knees, ankles or joints.

* **Make Exercise Fun**: There are going to be days when doing any exercise at all feels like too much effort. The trick is to figure out ways to make your exercise as much fun as possible so that you will want to do it on days when you aren't feeling motivated. Dancing is one of the more fun ways to exercise. Today there are lots of innovative dance classes, and the best part is once you learn the routines you can put on some music do them at home. Think of your exercise as a gift that you give to yourself. Who wouldn't want a present that helps you stay in shape and feel great all at the same time?

De-Stress to be Your Best

Stress is not necessarily a bad thing and our bodies are designed to handle a certain amount of stress. For example, if you step off a curb and a car comes speeding towards you, your body responds in a way to help you react. At the outset of an event that causes stress, your body will have a physical reaction, such as shallow breathing or a feeling that your heart is racing. This triggers the release of two hormones: adrenalin and cortisol. In a stressful situation, cortisol quickly breaks down available sugars, fats & proteins in order to supply energy so that you can get out of the way of the car coming towards you. Then, once the "crisis" is over the body returns to normal.

Unfortunately, in today's world we experience "Chronic Stress" from all directions, including finances, career, deadlines, lack of time, family, the environment and world events. Our bodies can't tell the difference between stress from a car speeding towards you and the stress you feel when bills are late. When stress is ongoing, here is what happens:

Cortisol tries to supply energy. But, if you are constantly feeling stressed out and there is no ready supply of protein available, then cortisol begins to steal nitrogen from the structural protein in our muscles. It converts the protein to sugar for energy, and the end result is the ongoing destruction of the muscle needed to burn fat. When stress is a constant, and continues unmanaged, this process repeats itself over and over again.

Ongoing stress increases carbohydrate cravings & decreases serotonin levels, causing you to crave sweets and carbohydrates Over time, the effects of chronic stress and high levels of cortisol include: Loss of Muscle Tissue, Stress Eating, Erratic/High Blood Sugars, Excess Insulin Production, Fat Storage, Fatigue, and Chronic Illness Additionally, losing muscle mass is a major problem if you are trying to lose weight, because fat is burned within our muscle cells for energy. The more muscle you carry the more fat you can burn for energy, and studies show that losing even 1 ounce of muscle mass lowers the body's ability to create energy and reduces your fat burning ability.

Bottom Line: The combination of being in a constant state of stress + high glycemic carbohydrates results in more fat storage with a decreased ability to lose it as high cortisol levels diminish your ability to burn fat!

To maintain health, de-stressing is not a luxury, it is a necessity. Stress is a part of modern life. But, you can develop daily success habits to manage stress, including:

❖ Practice Deep Breathing: accessing the lower portion of your lungs activates a relaxation response in our bodies

❖ Incorporate at least ½ hour of a de-stressing activity into your daily routine (deep breathing, yoga, meditation, massage, etc.)

❖ Make your health a priority, and take some time for yourself every day.

❖ Exercise (walking, running, etc) for at least ½ hour 5-7 days a week.

❖ Write in a journal.

❖ Practice Gratitude & Enjoy Life!

❺ Find Out Where You Are & Monitor Your Progress

In order to stay on track with your program, it is important to take stock of where you are on a routine basis. Here are some of the important ways that you will want to monitor your ongoing progress.

Checkups and Testing:

Make sure to schedule regular checkups with your health care providers, and to keep up with physical exams and testing as outlined in the Diabetes Primer. As a reminder, here are some of the key areas that you want to keep up with on a regular basis.

❖ Fasting Glucose Levels

❖ HBA1C Test

❖ Lipid Profile

❖ Homocysteine Levels

❖ C-Reactive Protein

❖ Blood Pressure Monitoring

❖ Eye Exams

❖ Foot Exams

❖ Dental Exams and Routine Dental Care

❖ Thyroid Testing (Levels of T_4 and T_3 thyroid hormones in your blood

Daily Glucose Monitoring

For many new diabetics, pricking themselves to monitor their blood sugars is a scary prospect. For some it brings home the reality of being diabetic, and so they avoid it.

But, monitoring your blood sugar levels on a daily basis is a critical part of your program. Keeping tight glucose control involves monitoring your blood with a glucose meter. Based on results, you can quickly adjust diet, exercise or medication to keep your blood glucose levels within an acceptable range. If you are feeling hesitant about using a glucose monitor, seek the assistance of a health care provider who can show you how to use it.

The objective of daily monitoring is to keep your blood glucose under tight control and as close to normal as possible. Research shows that maintaining good glucose control on a daily basis can pay big dividends in avoiding diabetic complications later on.

📖 *Reflections*

When I was first diagnosed with diabetes I was "petrified" of testing my blood sugars. So, I asked my husband if he would prick his finger with the lancing device, and if it didn't hurt, then I would try it. Without hesitation, he did it and smiled up at me and said "no problem, hon." I've been testing my blood sugars 4 times a day ever since, and looking back it is hard to believe I was so frightened. Far from being a burden, knowing I can test myself, and make needed adjustments has given me both a feeling of freedom and .control, and testing has been an enormous help in letting my understand what foods I want to include in my food plan.

When to Test: The number of times you test yourself daily varies based on your condition. But, the goal should be to test yourself enough so that you have the information you need on a daily basis to adjust your food plan, exercise routine and medication in order to keep your blood glucose levels under control. Although there are no hard and fast rules on when to test, there are some generally accepted standard times to test These can include:

❖ Before breakfast, (fasting)

❖ Two hours after breakfast, lunch, dinner and large snacks

❖ One Hour after a meal or snack, (occasionally)

This can be helpful if you are in a period where your blood sugars are running higher than your norm or if you are trying to ascertain the effect of a particular food on your blood sugar levels. What you will discover by testing both an hour and then two hours after a meal is how long after a meal your highest reading comes... and how fast you return to "normal." Also, you may learn that a meal that included bread, fruit or other starches and sugars gives you a higher reading.

❖ Before and/or after exercise

❖ Before bedtime, occasionally

❖ At 2 A.M. or 3 A.M. occasionally (helpful if you are experiencing the "dawn effect" with higher blood sugar readings in the morning.

You should discuss your testing needs with your physician to determine the schedule that is best suited for your particular needs. One important word of advice: keep your testing results in perspective. The purpose of the testing is to give you feedback so that you can take action to improve the results if they are not within acceptable ranges.

Here are what doctors currently believe to be non-diabetic readings:

❖ Fasting blood sugar under 100 mg/dl (5.5 mmol/L)

❖ One hour after meals under 140 mg/dl (7.8 mmol/L)

❖ Two hours after meals under 120 mg/dl (6.6 mmol/L)

At a minimum, The American College of Clinical Endocrinologists recommends that people with diabetes keep their blood sugars under 140 mg/dl two hours after eating.

People ask me all the time whether they can eat certain foods. For example, because they are such popular foods, I get a lot of questions about breakfast foods like Cheerios and bananas. No matter what I advise or what any expert tells you, if you test your blood sugars and a food raises your blood sugar over the targets you are aiming for, that food should not be part of your diabetes food plan. So, although I generally recommend avoiding ripe bananas and refined cereals, the real test is how your own body responds. Remember that everyone's biochemistry is different, and ultimately, your blood sugar meter (along with your routine HbA1c screening) will tell you what the best "diabetes food plan" is for your body.

Do not judge yourself harshly. If you find yourself off-track or you are having trouble keeping your glucose levels under control, seek assistance from your health care team. They will be able to guide you in adjusting your food and exercise plan and can help you determine if additional medications or changes in medications are necessary. Be confident and know that if you get back to basics, your glucose levels will improve.

HbA1c Screening Test

In addition to daily monitory, getting an HbA1c test every 3-4 months will help you to see how you are doing over a period of time. This blood test indicates your average blood glucose over a 2-3 month period. ***It is not a substitute for daily glucose monitoring***, which is an important aspect of glucose control. Studies show that people with diabetes who keep their HBA1C levels below 7% are less likely to have diabetic complications. An HBA1C reading of 5%, indicates an average blood glucose level of 80, a reading of 6% indicates an average blood glucose level of 115, 7% indicates an average blood glucose level of 150, and 8% indicates an average blood glucose level of 180.

Using a Daily Journal

When you begin to use a journal on a daily basis you make a written commitment to yourself to alter your habits and make healthy changes in your lifestyle. Study after study has found that journaling is a powerful tool that you can use to brainstorm, track your progress and help you to keep moving forward towards your goals. Keeping a daily journal is a process that is designed to:

❖ Raise your awareness about what you eat on a daily basis and help you to avoid unconscious eating,

❖ Reinforce successful eating habits so that they become a natural part of your routine,

❖ Uncover your particular eating patterns so that you can take responsibility for your nutritional lifestyle, and

❖ Enable you to make the connection between the habits you build on a daily basis, (including exercise and food intake) and your ability to control your blood sugar levels.

If you are vigilant in tracking your progress, you will see patterns of behavior emerge, and you will gain a better understanding of how to develop and maintain success habits that support your ability to lose weight and manage your blood sugars.

As you begin to assimilate success habits into your daily routine, you may find that you don't need to use a journal everyday. But, you can always come back to it during times of stress or periods where you need extra help to keep on track. For optimum results:

❖ At the beginning of the week set forth the activities that you will commit to in furtherance of your goals. Determine a reward that you may receive if you meet your commitment(s). At the end of the week, note if you were able to meet you commitments, and if not, take time to reflect on what issues came up for you.

❖ Each day, track the food you are consuming.

❖ Note when you consume your food (Breakfast, Lunch, Dinner, Snack.) If you are diabetic, this will enable you to correlate the consumption of foods with any blood glucose results that are higher than desired.

❖ If you are diabetic, monitor your blood glucose levels noting the result and time of testing.

❖ Each day, incorporate an activity to reduce your stress level.

❖ Keep track of the amount of water or tea consumed.

❖ Note the amount of time you spend exercising. (Walking, jogging, aerobics, etc.)

Be as accurate as possible with what you eat and the amount. Portion sizes are important, but do not get hung up on precision measurements. The idea is to track what types of foods you are eating so that you can develop the habit of eating foods that support your ability to lose weight and control your blood sugar levels. The type of journal you use will depend on your personality and what works best for you.

The Great Life Daily Journal, is available through www.diabetescoaching.com by filling in the contact information and indicating that you would like to have an electronic version of the journal sent to you.

Below are some ideas for how to set your weekly goals.

Weekly: Goals & Intentions:

Activity Commitments:

First, identify 3 activities that you can commit to during the week that will lead you towards your health goals. The goals may vary from week to week depending upon the state of your health and the challenges you are facing.

Examples:

- ❖ Walk for 20 minutes at least 5 days
- ❖ Eliminate flour and eat only sprouted grain bread
- ❖ Add one new vegetable to evening meal

Obstacles:

Next, identify any obstacles you might encounter? Thinking ahead will help you to be prepared and in a better position to meet your goals. What ideas come to mind that will help you to overcome these obstacles?

Goal Review:

At the end of the week, note whether you were able to keep your commitments during the week. The purpose of noting whether you met your goals is to think about what came up for you and to give yourself the space to identify some action steps that will enable you to do things differently in the future. It is not about beating yourself up.

Be gentle with yourself, and remember that you can always adjust your strategy to get back on track.

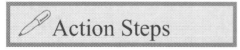 Action Steps

- ❖ Monitor your blood sugar levels per the instructions in this section.
- ❖ Set weekly goals and intentions (print and use the Weekly Goal sheet below)
- ❖ Use a Daily Journal (print and use the Daily Journal page set forth following the goal sheet or download the Daily Journal at www.diabetescoaching.com

WEEK: GOALS AND INTENTIONS

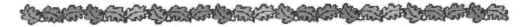

Live your life each day as you would climb a mountain. An occasional glance toward he summit keeps the goal in mind, but many beautiful scenes are to be observed from each new vantage point. Climb slowly, steadily, enjoying each passing moment; and the view from the summit will serve as a fitting climax for the journey.

Harold B. Melchart

Activity Commitments

Identify 3 activities that you can commit to this week that will lead you towards your health goals:

OBSTACLES

Identify any obstacles you might encounter? What are some ideas for what you might do to overcome these obstacles:

I kept my commitments this week: ☐ Yes ☐ No

If no, what are some thoughts on what you might be able to do differently in the future?

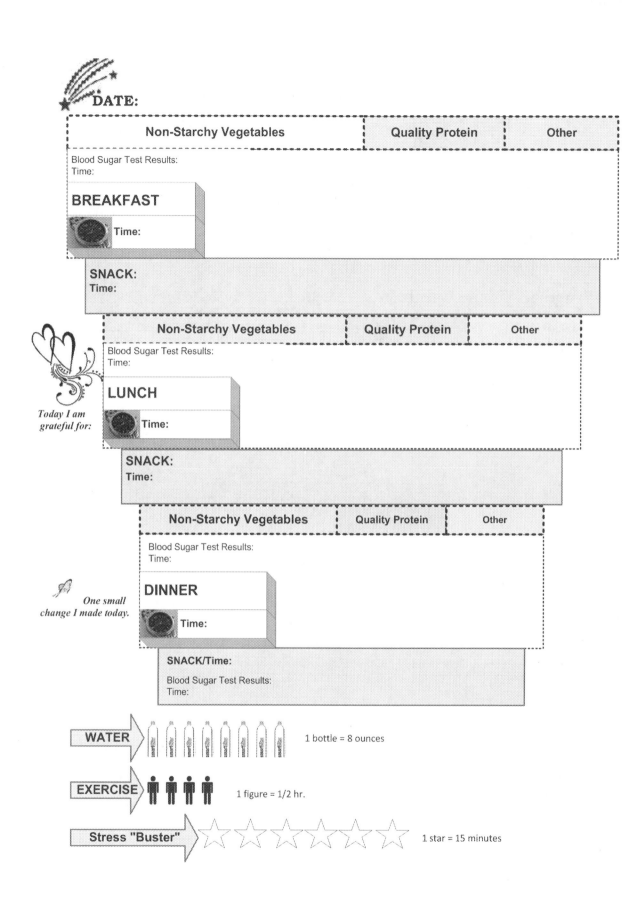

DATE:

Non-Starchy Vegetables	Quality Protein	Other

Blood Sugar Test Results:
Time:

BREAKFAST

Time:

SNACK:
Time:

Non-Starchy Vegetables	Quality Protein	Other

Blood Sugar Test Results:
Time:

LUNCH

Time:

Today I am grateful for:

SNACK:
Time:

Non-Starchy Vegetables	Quality Protein	Other

Blood Sugar Test Results:
Time:

DINNER

Time:

One small change I made today.

SNACK/Time:

Blood Sugar Test Results:
Time:

WATER — 1 bottle = 8 ounces

EXERCISE — 1 figure = 1/2 hr.

Stress "Buster" — 1 star = 15 minutes

❻ Reverse Behaviors that are Sabotaging your Health

Conquering a chronic condition like diabetes is not easy, especially when you are trying to change familiar routines and behaviors that no longer serve your best interests.

Most people can stick to a new plan for a short period of time. It is the long haul that puts you to the test. So, how do you reverse behaviors that sabotage your health for the long term? The trick is to:

- ❖ Make your conquer diabetes plan a priority,
- ❖ Make daily choices that support your vision of health, and
- ❖ Make the most of your time and energy.

For many people, making themselves a priority is incredibly difficult. Chronic illness is often a sign that you are out of balance, stretched too thin and need to take the focus off others and put it on yourself.

Many people are afraid to pay too much attention to their own needs out of a fear that they will appear "selfish", especially where friends and family are concerned. To the contrary, what could be more giving than making the effort to become healthy so that you can be there for your friends and family as a stronger person able to participate more fully in life?

An important part of investing in yourself is making choices that support your vision of health. In addition to what you will eat, how often you will exercise, and what medications or supplements you will take, these lifestyle choices include how you will spend your time and even how you will manage your finances to purchase items that you need to manage your condition.

When it comes to things like eating fresh vegetables, taking supplements, attending a workshop or even conducting daily monitoring (which requires testing supplies), it is not uncommon for individuals to come to the conclusion that they cannot afford these "luxuries." Financial issues are a reality. But, if you find yourself using money as a reason not to pursue an activity that could help you, take the time to explore all of your options. When you really want something, it is amazing what the universe provides.

📖 *Reflections*

Like a lot of people with diabetes, I have children, a job, friends, and they all seem to require a good deal of my time and attention. When I first began to get my blood sugars under control, it was difficult to say no to requests or invitations when I needed time to rest, exercise or prepare dishes for my food plan.

But one thing was clear in my mind...every minute my blood sugars were high was a minute that damage was being done to my body. So for me the choices were clear, and I did my best to strike a balance in terms of still being there for the people in my life. Ironically, as my blood sugars stabilized, I started feeling so much better that I had even more time than before to spend doing things with my family and friends, and I was able to function 100% better at work.

Changing Behavior: How to "STOP" repeating Habits that are Sabotaging Your Success

It is not unusual to have a strong desire to change a behavior, yet still find yourself repeating old patterns. **STOP** is a method that slows down the action so that you can step back and gain more clarity about the link between your thoughts, feelings and subsequent behaviors. This in turn allows you to get in touch with the inner voice that can guide you to making better choices. The next time you find yourself reaching for the cookie jar, skipping your exercise or eating half the bread basket, try the steps below.

Step Outside Yourself: When you are in the midst of a behavior that you know is sabotaging your health, literally take a break in the "action" and take a look at what you are doing as if you are an impartial observer. This does two things. First, it raises the level of your action from an "unconscious" behavior that is seemingly beyond your control to one that can be changed. Second, at a practical level it slows you down so that you can exercise some options.

> For example, let's imagine that at the end of a long work day you come through your front door and find yourself standing in front of an open cabinet, eating your way through a box of crackers. On auto-pilot, you just keep eating as if in a trance until you get to the end of the box.

Using the **STOP** method, the goal in this situation would be to consciously stop what you are doing for a moment so that you can set the stage for taking another course of action. Observe yourself right then as if you are a stranger watching a scene from a movie.

* What is your physical state? (how is your breathing, heartbeat, other physical sensations) Are you standing or sitting? Have you taken your coat off?
* Look at the crackers. What kind are they? How do they taste? Did you get a plate or are you just eating them quickly out of the box?

Now that you have slowed the action down you are ready to take the next step.

Trace Your Current Action Back to the "Triggering" Event. Think back on what occurred that got you to this point. In other words, as best as you can, trace your current action back to what I call the "triggering event.

> In this situation, let's imagine that you ate a healthy breakfast and lunch, and you had a small snack of nuts and low-fat cheese around 3:00. So as you reflect upon the situation, physically, there is no reason for you to be ravenous.
>
> Thinking back, you remember that your boss took credit for some work that you did. (This is something that happens on a pretty regular basis, not just to you but to everyone in the department.) But, you didn't say anything about it. Instead, you "stewed" about it all afternoon and by the time you got home your emotions were "eating away at you".

Tracing your current action back to events that "stimulated" your current action is crucial because it enables you uncover what is motivating your behavior and to clarify your thinking. It is a powerful technique that creates the opportunity to ask yourself questions that will reveal whether your behavior is in your best interest and to brainstorm about new behaviors that can be put its place.

Observe Your Thoughts and Clarify Your Actions. Bringing conscious awareness to our choices enables us opens the door to an honest self-assessment where we can ask ourselves questions that will clarify the consequences of our actions. Through this process, we gain clarity about the choices we make and whether our actions support or sabotage our vision of health and well-being.

In this case if you are able to see that you were angry and were attempting to push your feelings down with food, you are in a better position to make a change in your behavior so that you can learn to address anger in a way that does not involve compulsive eating.

- ❖ Is the action of compulsive eating an action that is a helpful behavior to deal with your anger?
- ❖ What are the positive aspects of using food to calm yourself down?
- ❖ What are the costs to you and your overall health?
- ❖ Does compulsive eating at the end of a work day lead you towards or away from your goals?

Mindless eating at the end of a long work day is actually quite common, although the triggering event varies based on individual circumstances. For some of my clients, reaching for comfort foods at the end of the work day is the result of not eating enough during the day. For others, it is a longstanding unconscious reaction to feelings such as boredom or anxiety. Regardless of the circumstances, once you can step back and identify the root causes and the choices you made in response to the circumstance, you are ready to take action steps to make a change.

Put a New Behavior in Place of the Old Behavior. The ultimate goal is to get yourself off of "auto-pilot" and to gain clarity about the choices you are making on a daily basis so that you can replace sabotaging habits with new behaviors. Just as you used empowering questions to identify activities that you could put in place to reach your goals, you can use the technique of asking targeted questions to regain your power over how you react to situations and your subsequent behaviors. The idea is to brainstorm to come up with alternative behaviors so that you will have options as to how you choose to react in the future to situations in a way that supports your well-being. In the situation where you are eating as a response to feeling angry, some empowering questions might be:

- ❖ **What can I do to deal with my anger in a way that does not harm me**? (Get up from my desk and take a walk, find a quiet spot to do some deep breathing, share my feelings with a trusted person, or write in a journal.)
- ❖ **What can I do to make sure that I have something healthy and ready to eat in the event that I am not feeling 100 percent when I get home from work**? (Shop on Sundays and keep healthy food choices easily accessible.- Examples: cut up vegetables and hummus, salad with condiments, roasted sliced chicken breast, low fat cheese, vegetable soup.)
- ❖ **What can I do to resolve my issues around emotional eating**? (Seek assistance from a therapist or life coach, write in my journal, or explore beliefs that may be at the core of my emotional eating)

NOW, close your eyes and visualize yourself doing the new behavior. How does it feel?

Finally, select some of the new behavior alternatives and practice putting them into place.

You may not be able to control the behaviors of others, but you can control your reactions and the choices you make that will ultimately either sabotage your efforts or lead you towards better health. With repetition, you will internalize new behaviors, and with practice they will eventually become automatic. Changing your lifestyle is not easy, but it is important to focus on what you can control and letting go of what you cannot.

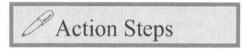 Action Steps

Conquer Emotional and Mindless Stress Eating:

For a huge number of people, the everyday act of eating is an overwhelming process. Have you ever wondered why this is so?

The sensations and emotions that signal when you are full, hungry or just wanting to eat something like candy, ice cream or potato chips is the result of a complex combination of chemical reactions occurring in our bodies along with emotional feelings.

If emotional eating (or eating in response to stress) is a strong factor affecting your eating behaviors, you may want to explore long standing beliefs underlying your actions and how you can change those beliefs in order to successfully change behaviors holding you back.

The key to changing the way you eat is not to become more disciplined by counting calories or going on a strict "diet", but learning how to master control of your mind.

This subject is beyond the scope of this workbook. But a good place to start is with the book "**The Power of Belief**" by Ray Dodd which explores these concepts in detail and provides a step by step program for gaining awareness so that you can transform your belief system to support personal growth.

Several additional books focusing on emotional and stress eating are listed in the "Suggested Reading and Resources" section.

❼ Establish Your Ongoing Support Team

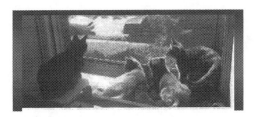

The diagnosis of diabetes or pre-diabetes turns your life upside down. Denial or ignoring the diagnosis can result in extremely serious consequences, and for this reason, the need to take action is fairly immediate. **Going it alone is not an option**. At a minimum, you will need the supervision of a family physician or diabetes specialist, typically an endocrinologist, to help you keep your glucose levels under control.

Other members of your support team depend on your particular needs. A diabetes coach can work with you to establish goals, provide practical tips for staying on track as well as help you to stay motivated as you implement your diabetes management program. The diagram below sets forth the types of professionals or support groups you might enlist to assist you reach your goals.

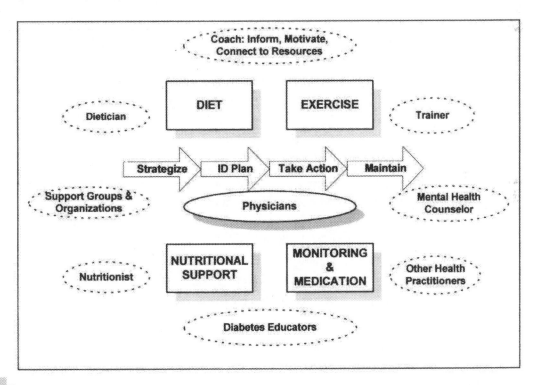

🔑 **Place yourself under the care of a physician you can talk to**: Let your physician know that you want to take an active role in your recovery, and that in addition to medications that the physician may recommend, you want to explore options relating to nutrition, exercise and helpful supplements. Most physicians will be very happy to help you to participate in your diabetes care. But, unfortunately, not all physicians are as open or as experienced as you need them to be when it comes to treating diabetes. If you really like your physician, try to work it out. If you can't, it is OK to find a physician that you feel more comfortable with.

❽ Enjoy Life

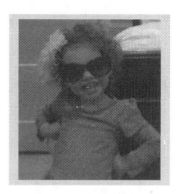

It is a real art to learn how to take care of a diabetic or pre-diabetic condition without letting it overtake all of your thoughts and energy. Getting through each day without thinking about your blood sugars at every waking moment is where success habits come in.

Remember, habits are repeated behaviors that ultimately become automatic. In the beginning, you need to put a lot of time, effort and thought into remembering to eat certain foods, to drink more water, to test your blood glucose, and to fit in exercise. But, as you practice these behaviors, over time they will become part of you, as much as brushing your teeth has become part of your routine over the years.

When you brush your teeth, you don't dwell on gum disease or the bad things that could happen if you don't take care of your teeth. You don't get upset or angry because you have to take a few minutes to indulge in some dental hygiene. Think of all the things you do every day, almost without any thought.

Taking care of yourself in a new way is challenging, and that is why in the beginning you need to pay more attention. Whether you choose to drain your mental energy by thinking negatively about changing your lifestyle is totally within your control. When you find it difficult to feel positively about doing "one more thing" to control your blood glucose levels, take a minute to recall your vision of health.

It may be hard to imagine now, but you will find that exercising success habits that support your ability to control your blood glucose levels are a reward unto themselves. It's a self-perpetuating cycle. The better you start to feel, the more you will want to do the things that move you towards your vision and help you feel better.

After a while, the habits that support blood sugar control will become as automatic as brushing your teeth. You will find your mind dwelling less on the fact that you have diabetes and your focus shifting to your overall well-being.

You will incorporate success habits such as taking a morning walk, asking the waiter not to bring bread to the table, skipping the sugary desserts, keeping a bottle of water with you, and performing your blood sugar monitoring all without the relentless voice in your head going on and on about your diabetes or pre-diabetes.

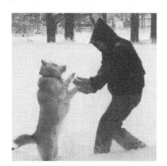

In short, you will begin to enjoy your life again.

In fact, there is no need to wait to begin enjoying your life. Do it now, even as you begin to implement your plan.

Have fun, and remember to incorporate little luxuries into every aspect of your day.

1. Wake up early and spend some quiet time meditating or writing in your journal.

2. Take a Walk. It doesn't have to be aerobic. Enjoy nature and your surroundings.

3 Have lunch with a friend, enjoy good conversation and fine food.

4. Cook up a perfect pot of chili and invite some friends over for supper.

5. BREATHE…

7. Light a scented candle, grab a good book and luxuriate in a good cup of tea. Green tea is especially beneficial for your overall health.

6. Take a Yoga Class.

Uncontrolled stress raises your cortisol levels, & can affect both your blood sugars and weight. Yoga is just one of many great ways to de-stress.

8. Concoct a magnificent sugar free dessert and share it with friends or family

9. Go dancing, it is a great way to get extra exercise

10. Get a massage or give one (both are fun).

15. MAKE YOUR WELL BEING A PRIORITY

You get the idea. Life is short. Diabetes or Pre-Diabetes only means that you are going to take care of yourself better than you ever have before. Dare to believe that you are going to enjoy yourself and live life to the fullest. What could be better than that?

11. Get a Coach. **Coaching can help you to reach your goals by providing guidance, ongoing support, motivation, and connection to resources.**

14. Take a personal day and do whatever comes to mind. Let the day take you wherever it leads.

12. Go to a movie, and don't forget to bring a delicious snack that you can enjoy during the previews.

13. Browse through the bookstore. Treat yourself to a new cookbook

16. Enjoy a GREAT LIFE.

☎ **610-642-3596**
✉ **janet.sanders@earthlink.net**
💻 **www.diabetescoaching.com**